Medical Biotechnology Innovation in India

This book examines the medical biotechnology industry in India through the lens of a critical political economy. It discusses the sharp trajectory of growth in the biotechnology business and the state of investments, subsidies, and patents which propelled the rise of the industry in India.

The book uses in-depth interviews and case studies to analyse the roles of various financial actors, state institutions, and academia in the medical biotechnology ecosystem. Focusing on the relationship between India's neoliberal policies and the swift growth of the industry, the author examines the merits and demerits of the current market-driven biomedical ecosystem exploring the trends in the industry, biomedical start-ups, the use of human resources, and capital accumulation process. The book reiterates and emphasises the need for the democratisation of scientific and medical work and for striking a balance between economic gains and public health priorities.

Comprehensive and insightful, this book will be of interest to scholars and researchers of science technology society studies, public health, economics, business studies, medical sociology, public policy, and political science.

P. Omkar Nadh is currently a postdoctoral researcher at the Indian Institute for Human Settlements, Bengaluru. He has a PhD from the Institute for Social and Economic Change, Bengaluru, and is a recipient of the Indian Council for Social Science Research fellowship.

Medical Biotechnology Innovation in India

A Critical Analysis

P. Omkar Nadh

Routledge
Taylor & Francis Group

LONDON AND NEW YORK

First published 2022
by Routledge
4 Park Square, Milton Park, Abingdon, Oxon OX14 4RN

and by Routledge
605 Third Avenue, New York, NY 10158

Routledge is an imprint of the Taylor & Francis Group, an informa business

© 2022 P Omkar Nadh

The right of P Omkar Nadh to be identified as authors of this work has been asserted in accordance with sections 77 and 78 of the Copyright, Designs and Patents Act 1988.

British Library Cataloguing-in-Publication Data
A catalogue record for this book is available from the British Library

Library of Congress Cataloging-in-Publication Data
A catalog record has been requested for this book

ISBN: 978-1-032-02214-7 (hbk)
ISBN: 978-1-032-27282-5 (pbk)
ISBN: 978-1-003-29210-4 (ebk)

DOI: 10.4324/9781003292104

Typeset in Sabon
by SPi Technologies India Pvt Ltd (Straive)

Contents

Illustrations

Figures

Tables

Abbreviations

ABI	Applied Biosystems Inc.
ABLE	Association for Biotechnology Led Enterprises
AUTM	Association of University Technology Managers
ARCI	Astra Research Centre India
ARIIA	Atal Ranking of Institutions on Innovation Achievements
BBC	Bangalore Bio Centre
BLiSC	Bangalore Life Science Cluster
BPAC	Bangalore Political Action Committee
BIBICOL	Bharat Immunological and Biological Corporation Limited
BCIL	Biotechnology Industry Consortium Limited
BIRAC	Biotechnology Industry Research Assistance Council
BIFR	Board for Financial and Industrial Reconstruction
CBT	Centre for Biotechnology
CCMB	Centre for Cellular and Molecular Biology
C-CAMP	Centre for Cellular and Molecular Platforms
CMS	Chatterjee Management Services
CRO	Clinical Research Organisation
CAGR	Composite Annual Growth Rate
CAG	Comptroller and Auditor General
CII	Confederation of Indian Industries
CSIR	Council for Scientific and Industrial Research
DBF	Dedicated biotech firm
DBT	Department of Biotechnology
DST	Department of Science and Technology
EY	Ernst & Young
FICCI	Federation of Indian Chambers of Commerce and Industry
FDA	Food and Drug Administration
FDI	Foreign Direct Investment
FVCIs	Foreign Venture Capital Investors
FITT	Foundation for Innovation and Technology Transfer
TCGA	The Centre for Genomic Applications
GoI	Government of India
GDP	Gross Domestic Product

HGP	Human Genome Project
IBEF	India Brand Equity Foundation
ICMR	Indian Council for Medical Research
IISc	Indian Institute of Science
IISER	Indian Institute of Science Education and Research
IIT	Indian Institute of Technology
IPCL	Indian Petrochemicals Corporation Limited
IVOCOL	Indian Vaccine Corporation Limited
IVCA	Indian Venture Capital Association
ICICI	Industrial Credit and Investment Corporation of India
IFCI	Industrial Finance Corporation of India
IDBI	Industrial Development Bank of India
IT	Information Technology
IPO	Initial Public Offering
ICT	Institute for Chemical Technology
IGIB	Institute for Genomics and Integrative Biology
IMM	Institute of Molecular Medicine
IPVE	Institute of Poliomyelitis and Viral Encephalitis
IIC	Institutional Innovation Council
IPTeL	Intellectual Property and Technology Licensing
IUPAC	International Union for Pure and Applied Chemistry
IVCs	International Value Chains
MBT	Medical Biotechnology
MoU	Memorandum of Understanding
M&A	Merger and Acquisition
MHRD	Ministry of Human Resource Development
NBTB	National Biotechnology Board
NBDS-I	National Biotechnology Development Strategy-I
NCBS	National Centre for Biological Sciences
NIH	National Institutes of Health
NIRF	National Institution Ranking Framework
NKC	National Knowledge Commission
NRDC	National Research Development Corporation
NPIL	Nicholas Piramal India Limited
NGO	Non-governmental Organisation
OPV	Oral Polio Vaccine
PMSV	Pasteur and Merieux Serum and Vaccines
PM	Prime Minister
PID	Product and Industry Development
PFRLs	Publicly Funded Research Laboratories
rDNA	recombinant DNA
R&D	Research and Development
S&T	Science & Technology
SEBI	Security and Exchange Board of India
SIDBI	Small Industries Development Bank of India

SID	Society for Innovation and Development
SBH	State Bank of Hyderabad
SBI	State Bank of India
SLiSc	Strand Life Sciences
TCGLS	TCG Lifesciences Pvt Ltd
TBIs	Technology Business Incubators
TDB	Technology Development Board
TTOs	Technology Transfer Offices
TCGD	The Chatterjee Group Developments India Pvt Ltd
TRIPS	Trade-Related Intellectual Property Rights Agreement
UTI	Unit Trust of India
UK	United Kingdom
US	United States
UGC	University Grants Commission
USD	US dollars
USPTO	US Patent and Trademark Office
VCFs	VC funds
VC	Venture Capital
WB	World Bank
WTO	World Trade Organisation
WW-II	World War II

Acknowledgements

The work presented in this book is largely a part of my doctoral dissertation that I carried out at the Institute for Social and Economic Change (ISEC), Bengaluru. Numerous people have helped in this process, and I would like to take this opportunity to thank at least a few of them. Firstly, I would like to thank my family for being a constant source of support and strength. I am also deeply indebted to my PhD advisor Dr. Sobin George for the many unending discussion sessions, critical inputs, and emotional support. Thanks also to my doctoral committee members Dr. Anil Kumar, Dr. Sunandan, and Dr. Bitasta Das and Prof. Supriya RoyChowdary for their support and encouragement in this process. I am extremely grateful to the administrative staff and contractual workers at ISEC for ensuring a space that helped me with the completion of this dissertation. I would also like to thank the Indian Council for Social Science Research for the fellowship provided for three years. I am also very grateful to all my respondents for giving me their valuable time during my fieldwork. My current workplace, the Indian Institute for Human Settlements, has extended great support in completing this manuscript. Special thanks to Gautham Bhan for being a source of encouragement and for providing me with valuable inputs to improve the manuscript. Parts of Chapter 1 will appear as a journal article in the *East Asian Science Technology Society Studies: An International Journal* and Chapter 4 in the journal *Social Science Information*.

My friends and comrades from ISEC and the University of Hyderabad have been a great source of strength in my journey, and I would like to thank all of them. Thanks also to Dr. Shoma Choudhary, commissioning manager, Routledge India, for ensuring a smooth flow of process and extending help to be able to successfully complete this manuscript. Finally, thanks to the anonymous reviewers for their invaluable suggestions.

Omkar

Capitalism, Neoliberalism, and Biotechnology

Neoliberalism as a dominant form of political-economic practice started gaining prominence during the late 1970s and early '80s as a result of an ongoing economic crisis that manifested during that period. One of the core tenets of the neoliberal theory that became a basis for its praxis is that markets are best suited to ensure efficient allocation of resources maximising the interests of the society as a whole. The role of the state, according to this theory, is to be less intervening in markets and take a back seat in ensuring social welfare measures. The theory advocates, left on their own, that individuals maximise their interests in a marketplace without any necessary role of the state (Navarro, 2007). The rationale behind such a reduced role of the state is that it distorts market signals and thereby accords wrong prices. Adopting these ideas, most states across the globe have undergone neoliberalisation by deregulating their markets, ensuring large-scale privatisation, and withdrawing from social welfare (Harvey, 2005). However, the practice of neoliberalism has deviated from its theoretical position in one of the most fundamental aspects. Under the guidance of the neoliberal theory, while states have largely withdrawn themselves from social welfare thinking that markets are in a better position to ensure the well-being of all, in sharp contrast, they have actually intervened in markets in the interest of a small section of the business class by providing various incentives such as capital support through public-private partnerships (PPPs), access to several public resources at below-market or no price, and various forms of tax breaks. This deviation from the stated theory to practice according to Harvey (ibid., p. 16) is because the project of neoliberalisation is also a "political project to re-establish the conditions for capital accumulation and to restore the conditions of economic elites." Under such neoliberal practice, institutions that were imagined to be governed by an egalitarian ethic started transforming championing the cause of private capital accumulation while at the same time shedding from their social role.

It was during the same period of the emergence of neoliberalism as the guiding principle of political-economic practice that a sub-discipline in the academic field of life sciences called biotechnology came into prominence that soon transformed into an industry. Biotechnology is a techno-scientific

DOI: 10.4324/9781003292104-1

advancement ushered with an epistemological shift in the field of life sciences that was attempting to understand the basis of life at a micro-scale/ molecular level. This attribution of techno-scientific idiosyncrasy to biotechnology stems from the fact that it simultaneously attempts to understand the basis of life biologically at the micro-level, and at the same time develops tools to address any abnormalities that deviate from this new micro-level normal. Before the emergence of this micro-level understanding of biological life in life sciences, what was prevalent was a dual category of the body for medical intervention in terms of "the normal" and "the pathological" captured by the clinical gaze (Foucault, 2003). This distinction collapsed with the advancement of microbiology and in turn gave rise to a new normal[1] and a spectrum of pathologies (Rose, 2001). The spectrum of pathologies provided scope for a wide range of interventions through a variety of tools under the ambit of what is commonly referred to as MBT. Further, the arising of new possibilities to biologically intervene in bettering life gave rise to an economic opportunity resulting in the emergence of an MBT industry often referred to as bioeconomy in policy circles. For instance, the Organisation for Economic Co-operation and Development (2009) defines bioeconomy as "the set of economic activities relating to the invention, development, production and use of biological products and processes." It is this entanglement of the "bio" with the "economic"—particularly in the context of MBT—under the neoliberal political-economic regime that is the subject matter of this book focusing on the Indian context. The book is specifically interested in teasing out the role of state, academia and fiancé capital in constituting a MBT ecosystem in India and examining the nature of their participation.

In the United States (US) where the biotech phenomenon first emerged, according to Melinda Cooper (2008, p.19), "the biotech revolution, (...), is the result of a whole series of legislative and regulatory measures designed to relocate economic production at the genetic, microbial, and cellular level, so that life becomes, literally, annexed within capitalist processes of accumulation." Further, it was also witnessed from the experience of the countries such as the US that, for the entanglement of the "bio" with the "economic" to take place, what was "vital" was the coming together of various actors and institutions—often referred to as ecosystem—particularly the state, academia, and the finance capital that were largely pursuing a conflicting set of agendas and interests before the occurrence of this phenomenon. As a result, particularly the state and academia had to shed their social roles and get appropriated in the interest of private capital accumulation. This becomes evident when one closely looks at the evolutionary trajectory of the MBT to which I move on to in the following section. The reason that I focus on the US is because it is the first country across the globe to have a successful MBT industry and as Birch (2006) points out, the US MBT industry attained some kind of a "mythical status" that drove policies in other countries.

MBT: A Brief History

The evolutionary history of MBT provides a sense of some of its significant milestones, and, in fact, in one sense, summarise the necessary historical details that are essential for the critical enquiry that this book engages with. As Pisano (2006) points out, MBT research, unlike previous applied research which guaranteed returns from the market, is the use of basic science[2] itself for economic value generation. He characterises this phenomenon as a '*science-based business*,' meaning it does not just attempt to use the existing scientific knowledge but also advances scientific knowledge and captures the economic value of such advancement. In the US, where the biotech phenomenon first emerged, while the overall federal funding for scientific research and development (R&D) declined with time, of this declined amount, institutions involved in biotechnology R&D were receiving close to 50% of the grants (AAAS, 2018). It was debates in MBT that led to the expansion of the ambit of patent laws to the extent of patenting life forms (Krimsky, 2003).The commercial establishment of MBT preceded a huge multinational co-operative effort in the form of the Human Genome Project (HGP).The commercial establishment of MBT is dovetailed with several new changes in the rules of the market game. It brought together several new actors with previously divergent functions and conflicting interests and institutionalised several new processes. The following sections discuss these milestones in further detail.

Science-Based Business

Historically, with the exception of a few big industries such as IBM, General Electric, and Xerox, science and business largely operated in separate spheres (Pisano, 2006). According to Pisano (2006), it was only with the advent of biotechnology that basic research started becoming a commercial endeavour. With basic science research taking a new commercial shape, so did the actors that were previously engaging with it. It was only the universities and academic spaces that were mostly pursuing basic research previously. With the advent of science-based business, basic science research ceased being an exclusive activity of universities and academia, as did business activities cease being limited only to commercially oriented firms. The universities and academic spaces started engaging in business activities while the commercial firms engaged in basic science research. There was an emergence of what is called an entrepreneurial university/venture science with some new additions and deletions to its existing structures (Etzkowitz, 2003; Sunder Rajan, 2012). A few notable changes to the structure of the university observed across the globe are as follows:

i.   The institutionalisation of Technology Transfer Offices (TTOs) that market university research.

ii. Universities spinning off start-ups for an equity stake.
iii. Scientists from the universities starting their own start-ups while also working as full-time members at the university.

All of these aforementioned characteristics can be demonstrated if one looks at the case of Genentech, a successful first-generation dedicated bio-tech firm (DBF) in the US. The demonstration of the case of Genentech also becomes important because this model is emulated by most DBFs across the globe and is followed till today.

The Story of Genentech

Genentech is a DBF established in the year 1972 by a university-based biochemist named Dr. Herbert Boyer and aspiring venture capitalist Robert Swanson. Boyer is one of the discoverers of the recombinant ribose nucleic acid (rDNA)[3] technology when he was a scientist at the University of Chicago, and this research was partly funded by pub-lic money (Hughes, 2001). After realising the commercial potential of this technology, he established Genentech. The founding of Genentech brought along with it certain changes to the academic scenario that existed till then. It was for the first time that a university faculty member started their own business establishment while also holding onto their position at the university (Hughes, 2011). Though patenting was hap-pening much before this, it was for the first time that basic science results were patented (ibid.). In fact, the discoverers took a long time to patent their research because of the then prevailing academic ethos where it was believed that basic science research knowledge should be free and public (ibid.). Stanley N. Cohen, who along with Boyer discovered rDNA technology, recollects in an interview that when he was approached by Niels Reimer who was the TTO officer at Stanford University for pat-enting rdna technology, his "framework was that one patents devices, not basic scientific methodologies" (Hughes, 2001, p. 549). However, the discovery of the rDNA method was patented at the insistence of the TTO from Stanford University in association with the University of California.[4] This event marked the beginning of the institutionalisation of licencing university research results in a way that commercialisa-tion became a priority for the university administration (Sunder Rajan, 2012). Such institutionalisation and normalisation that followed were looked at differently by various scholars. On one side of the spectrum were those who argued that, with the commercialisation of science, the pursuit of scientific knowledge had aligned more towards market needs rather than addressing the larger public good. Sunder Rajan (ibid., p. 3) articulates this phenomenon as, "the emergence of entrepreneurial university; the corporatisation of life sciences; the naturalisation of this corporatisation." On the other hand, Etzkowitz (2003) saw this process to be very normal and as just a continuation of what universities are supposed to evolve into. He, in fact, termed this change as a 'Second Academic Revolution,' with the first one being the addition of research to the teaching function of a university. After Genentech, this specific form of university-industry relation where universities and scientists acting entrepreneurially only got normalised, becoming an important component of the mode of production in the contemporary innovation-led bioeconomies. This addition of new actors and institutions previously not associated with the market and the normalisation of their participation into the market structure marks an important beginning in the historical trajectory of MBT.

The history of academia-industry in the US can be traced back to the period between World War I and World War II (WW-II), such as the ones between Eli Lilly, the multinational pharmaceutical firm, and the University of Toronto, and Eli Lilly and the University of Rochester in 1922 and 1931, respectively (Blumenthal, 2003). However, such relationships went on a decline once the large companies started in-house R&D and universities were supported by federal funding. A study by Blumenthal et al. (1986) finds that a revolution in biotechnology rejuvenated the industry's interest to establish a relationship with the university. At the beginning of the so-called biotech revolution, around one-third of the university's research was supported by the industry (Blumenthal, Gluck, Louis, & Wise, 1986). Stanford has become an exemplar of an entrepreneurial university, especially in the field of life sciences through the licencing of a patent on rDNA technology developed by Stanley Cohen and Herbert Boyer (Sunder Rajan, 2012). Though universities were performing sponsored projects before, with Stanford, what one has witnessed is an institutionalisation of commercialisation of basic research (ibid.). TTOs became an integral part of universities, and DBFs were also being spun out from the universities to commercialise their research. The nature of commercial relationships of university with industry are usually of many types, such as universities performing sponsored projects, universities licencing their patents and collaborative research by university and industry, consultation by members of faculty to industry, equity holding in companies by universities or faculties, and support of graduate students by companies. With the increasing commercialisation of knowledge, the boundaries between university and firm started blurring, and universities were increasingly being integrated into market structures. Particularly in the context of biotech, Pisano (2006, p. 2) explained it vividly as follows:

In numerous instances, the boundary between a university and a biotech firm is blurred. The founders of a substantial number of biotech firms include the professors (many of them world-renowned scientists) who invented the technologies that the startups licensed from the universities, often in return for an equity stake. These companies frequently maintain their links with the universities, working closely with faculty members and post-doctoral candidates on research projects, and sometimes using the university laboratories. In many instances, the founding scientists even retain their faculty posts.

A study by Blumenthal (2003), finds that from the mid to late 1990s, 90% of firms conducting research in life sciences had *some* type of relationship with a university and about one-quarter of life science faculty from universities in the US received support from industry for their research projects. Also, around the same time, 50% of life science faculties from universities acted as consultants for the industry, and 7% of them held equity in a company that was performing work related to them. In 1999, a survey showed that 68% of universities in Canada and the US held equity in companies that sponsored research for their faculties (Blumenthal, 2003).

This trend has only been increasing with time. Though federal funding is still a major source for university research, empirical evidence shows an increasing trend in the funding by the industry and the universities themselves. For instance, between 2007 and 2017, while the state, local agencies, and federal government funding for university research decreased by 10% and 13.8 %, respectively, universities and industry funding increased by 30.6% and 10.6%, respectively (AAAS, n.d.). While there was a decline in the share of federal funding, the life science disciplines received more than 50% of the total federal funding (ibid.). The previous statistics indicate an increase in the entrepreneurial orientation by universities since an increase in university expenditure is implicitly linked with the resources they generate by strategies such as licencing and other options. In 1994, data from the Association of University Technology Managers (AUTM) showed that 120 US universities spawned 175 spin-offs which have been increased across disciplines with 155 universities producing 655 spin-offs in 2012 with more than half of them focusing on life sciences (Huggett, 2014). Recent data shows that while the top schools recorded 93 life sciences start-ups, the number almost doubled to 182 in 2015 (Huggett, 2017). The universities have also realigned themselves to transfer technologies to start-ups through their TTOs (ibid.). Life sciences and biotechnology are particularly outdoing other segments in these new proactive measures by the university. Tables 0.1 and 0.2 provide an overview of the amount of revenues by technology transfers and spin-offs that universities have generated over five years (2011–2015) and how life sciences were dominating the whole scenario.

Table 0.1 Revenues Generated and Spin-Offs from Top Schools in the US between 2011 and 2015

S. No	University	Licence and/ or Options Executed	Gross Licencing Revenue ($)	Start-Ups
1	University of Washington	284	31,417,773	12
2	University of California System	248	169,724,803	66
3	University of Texas System	128	48,083,097	23
4	Stanford University	88	88,573,239	18
5	Columbia University	70	181,400,000	19
6	Massachusetts Institute of Technology	68	17,000,000	10
7	New York University	53	209,000,000	12
8	University of Utah	49	59,495,096	11
9	University of Massachusetts	24	31,814,000	4
10	Northwestern University	22	61,565,351	7
11	Princeton University	4	136,541,760	0

Source: Huggett (2017, p. 203)

Table 0.2 Comparison of Gross Revenues, Licences Executed, and Start-ups Formed by Top Universities in the US between 2011 and 2015

Licences/Options Executed		Gross Revenue ($)		Start-Ups Formed	
Overall	Life Sciences	Overall	Life Sciences	Overall	Life Sciences
1,471	1,038(70.56%)	1,106,458,949	1,034,615,079 (93.5%)	262	182 (69.46%)

Source: Huggett (2017, p. 203)

Budgetary Allocations for MBT R&D by the State: The US Experience

The research university as we know it today in the US was established during the last quarter of the 19th century, at about the same time as the establishment of the modern industrial corporation (National Science Foundation, 1982). Before the 1930s, university research was largely supported by private corporations and endowment funds from big philanthropic organisations such as the Rockefeller Foundation and the Carnegie Institution of Washington (National Science Foundation, 1982). During the post-war period (after the 1930s), this previously existing relationship between the university and industry gradually declined over a period of time, largely because of the Great Depression that took place then (National Science Foundation, 1982). Thereafter, the American state started playing a very prominent role in scientific research in universities. This can be explained by the fact that 73% of R&D expenditure at the universities was federally funded during the late 1960s in the US (AAAS, n.d.). However, from the early 1980s, there was a decline in state funding to university R&D (AAAS, n.d.). This was also the period during which President Ronald Regan started implementing neoliberal measures in the US. The decline in welfare measures, dilution of the trade union movement, implementation of austerity measures, and ensuring supply-side incentives were all witnessed during the same period (Cooper, 2008). Based on the same principle of incentivising the supply-side, although there was an overall decline in the federal funding of scientific research, out of the total funds allocated, nearly 50% was going to research in the areas of life sciences and biotechnology through institutions like the National Institute of Health (NIH; AAAS, 2018). While the US has provided increased budgetary support for life science research, during the same time, it has also enacted more than 15 legislations that allowed this publicly funded research to be transferred to private industry (Birch, 2006). Specifically, in the case of NIH, the enactment of the Stevenson Wydler Technology Innovation Act of 1980 has led to the creation of a TTO, as well as a separate centre for providing information to the private industry about commercialisable research (Birch, 2006).

The period also witnessed an increase in industry funding for university science and a substantial increase in revenues generated by the universities themselves with the rise of what is called an entrepreneurial university whose characteristics were described in the previous section. If one looks at the data with respect to discipline-wise funding from the state during the 1970s, total life sciences (including NIH funding) received close to 30%, whereas physical sciences and engineering received almost 50% of federal funding. By the beginning of the 1980s, life sciences received around 36%, while physical sciences and engineering received 41.7%. By the 1990s, life sciences were receiving around 41%, physical sciences and engineering were receiving close to 38% (AAAS, 2018). By 2003, life sciences started receiving more than 50% of the federal budget, while physical sciences and engineering received merely 26%. This trend carried from then on and in 2017, life sciences received around 50% of the federal budget (ibid.). What is important to note here is that it was during this period of increasing budgets in life sciences that the biotech phenomenon emerged in the US. During the same period, the rise of the entrepreneurial university was also witnessed, where universities were allowed to commercialise their federally funded research results, along with an increase in industry funding to university research. The industry-sponsoring university research increased by 20% higher than the overall average till then, and 50% of that increase was witnessed in biotechnology-related disciplines (Krimsky, 2003). All of these facts point to predominance of biotechnology and its increasing commercial status.

MBT, Multinational Co-operation, and the HGP

Another event that played a significant role in the commercial history of MBT was the HGP. HGP was a multinational co-operation project initiated by the US in 1990 with an estimated cost of three billion US dollars (USD) over a period of 15 years (National Human Genome Research Institute, n.d.). The project from the beginning was open to countries across the globe and by the end of the project, almost 18 countries participated in the project at different time points (Chial, 2008). However, the main participants were the US, the United Kingdom (UK), France, Germany, Japan, and China. The idea behind this mega project was to sequence the entire human genome so as to understand the underlying complex biological mechanisms of diseases that can help in the drug development process. A close look at the story of HGP reveals how this project was not just a scientific endeavour but one that is fraught with political and economic considerations. The project proposal was rejected initially by almost 80% of biologists along with the NIH (Hood & Rowen, 2013). It was the US Congress with its keen eye for international competitiveness in biology and medicine, potential for economic benefits, and industrial opportunities that gave an impetus to the project (Hood & Rowen, 2013). The reason for the initial reluctance from the scientific community was that such a mega exercise involving huge sums of money would dwarf the more essential small projects (Hood & Rowen, 2013). However, the project began in the year 1990, more at the insistence of the Department of Energy and the US Congress, later joined by the NIH (Hood & Rowen, 2013). The sequencing of the human genome presented itself with a myriad of possibilities commercially. It led to the rise of a commercial establishment that manufactures products which can put to use the data generated from HGP, annotate them, and decipher their functions and also tools and machinery that can be put to use in the project itself. One such tool that was widely spoken about was the high throughput sequencing machines manufactured by a company called Applied Biosystems Inc (ABI) (Sunder Rajan, 2006). ABI is a subsidiary of a company named Perkin-Elmer that was not so prominent till then and came into light only with the manufacture of sequence machinery. It also seeded another company named Celera Genomics, which was headed by Dr. Craig Venter. Dr. Venter worked at NIH till 1992 and left his position to head Celera Genomics later in 1999. After joining Celera Genomics, he challenged the public-funded HGP by announcing that they would sequence the genome before NIH and patent it. This created a kind of race between the two, with both of them finishing the sequencing almost closely behind each other and it is important to notice that the machines manufactured by ABI were needed for both of them to complete the project (Sunder Rajan, 2006). Once the sequencing was completed, the proponents of the project heralded it as a 'book of life,' 'code of codes,' etc. (Sunder Rajan, 2006) about the prospects that it had to offer. Finally, the multinational co-operation project aiming to address public health concerns was caught in a battle of 'public' versus 'private,' with the private agencies getting credit equal to the public ones (Sunder Rajan, 2006). Bill Clinton, the then president of the US, addressed the media with Dr. Venter and Dr. Francis Collins (head of NIH), announcing the successful sequencing of the human genome (Emmett, 2000). However, it was later realised that sequencing was just the beginning, and with the completion of HGP, a whole range of new commercial establishments and the beginning of what is called the post-genomic era started taking shape, putting to use the sequencing data generated by the HGP.

Patent Laws and MBT

Commercialisation of MBT while fuelled by the changes in the university structure and strong federal support, the dominant manifestation of this commercialisation takes place in the form of patents. Patents, as a reward system to the inventors, are not new to contemporary societies. As far back as in the 1200s, a ten-year monopoly was granted to inventors of a silk-making instrument in the city of Venice. Galileo was granted a patent by the Venetian state in 1594 for his invention of horse-driven water pumps (Krimsky, 2003). In 1624, England passed the Statute of Monopolies. Prior to the 1790s, American colonies were granted patents by special acts of colonial legislatures (Krimsky, 2003). In the 1790s, the US introduced in its Constitution, Article 1 Section 8, which states that "the Congress shall have the power to promote the progress of science and useful arts by securing for a limited time to authors and inventors the exclusive right to their respective writings and discoveries" (as cited in Krimsky, 2003, p. 59).

But what is more interesting in the contemporary bioeconomies is that patents have become so important that they form the nucleus of the innovation ecosystem. They derive monopoly rents for the DBFs that in a way became the defining objective of the existence of these firms (Birch, 2017). Even in the contemporary social practices of financial evaluation of biotech firms, patents occupy central stage. Particularly in the context of the bioeconomy, patents have acted as critical agents for the proliferation of the speculative business model. In the speculative business model, the prospective success of a firm is 'speculated' based on the number of patents that the firm has secured rather than the products or services developed by the firm.[5] Patents also played a crucial role in the emergence of the entrepreneurial university. The transformation in the contemporary academic value system is in a way fuelled, sustained, and ensured by the patent system since patents earn revenues for the universities through licencing and have become an integral part in evaluating the efficiency of scientists. While all of these are the effects of patents occupying the central stage in the MBT ecosystem, a crucial force behind this rapid transformation has been the legal pronouncement in the case of *Diamond* (Commissioner of Patents and Trademarks) *vs. Chakrabarty* in the US Supreme Court. This case, for the first time, legalised the patenting of life forms. Dr. Anand Chakrabarty, who was working for General Electric, discovered a soil micro-organism called Pseudomonas that can degrade an oil spill (Krimsky, 2003). Dr. Chakrabarty mixed different strains of Pseudomonas through genetic engineering for cleaning up spilled oil through degradation of hydrocarbons and filed a patent for the process of oil spilling and the living organism itself. The claim for the patent has been rejected by the US Patent and Trademark Office (USPTO) on the grounds that the bacteria is a natural and living organism. This decision was appealed at the Board of Appeals of the USPTO, and the board overturned the decision of USPTO that genetically modified bacteria was a product of nature; however, it still did not grant a patent to Dr. Chakrabarty on the grounds that living organisms are in and of themselves not patentable (Krimsky, 2003). The case then moved to the US Supreme Court where in a majority ruling of five to four, a patent was granted for the first time for a living organism. This case became a crucial force behind the proliferation of the MBT industry in the US by furthering the entanglement between the "bio" and the "economic". Before this judgement, patents were awarded only towards the outcomes and the processes that led to these outcomes. What this judgement essentially did was, it allowed owning any naturally occurring biological material provided they are sufficiently modified. This judgement also ended the ethical debate that was prevalent during that period with regard to owning life forms. To quote an industrial representative about the extent of impact the ruling has on the proliferation of biotech industry,

> Interestingly, before 1980, which is when the Supreme Court decision came out, there were only a handful of biotech companies. The innovator at the time was Genentech; then, after that, Cetus Chiron. But after Diamond v. Chakrabarty, the biotech industry grew phenomenally. Some say it is a coincidence, but I do not think so.
>
> (Feisee, 2002, p. 359)

MBT and the New Market Game

All of the aforementioned events are crucial in the trajectory of the commercial establishment of the MBT industry and towards understanding the role of political-economic actors behind the "bio" + "economic" entanglement. On the other hand, it was not just these events but several other market actors as well played a crucial role in the proliferation of the MBT industry. Most of the successful first-generation firms' business strategy was to come up with a patentable innovation and out-licence it to big pharma or look for a merger and acquisition (M&A) deal between both or go for an initial public offering (IPO). Not to forget that the drug development market space was previously entirely occupied by the pharmaceutical industry. It is important to note here that, during the same period of the rise of MBT, the pharmaceutical industry was also dealing with a potential crisis. This was largely due to the huge amount of capital investments and the high risk involved in the drug development process. The success rate in drug development is very abysmal and only one out of every five drugs that enter clinical trials is successful (Sunder Rajan, 2017). In addition, the industry was also dealing with the problem of the innovation cliff, where there is not enough patentable material in their pipelines (Sunder Rajan, 2017). However, around the same time, the development of disciplines like pharmacogenomics[6] helped the pharmaceutical industry in rationalising the drug development process. The situation has led the pharmaceutical industry to concede a little market space to the DBFs based on risk analysis. This led to a bifurcation in the terrain of drug development, with DBFs occupying the upstream terrain of R&D and pharmaceutical companies in the downstream taking these R&D results to manufacture drugs (Sunder Rajan, 2003). An important factor that helped establish this pattern of market structure is patent rights. Patent rights allow the DBFs to own the outcomes of their R&D and derive monopoly rents on it by out-licencing.

Another important economic actor that played a crucial role in the growth of commercial biotechnology is the venture capital (VC) industry. Again, the story of Genentech here provides some perspective. Along with Dr. Herbert Boyer, the co-founder of Genentech is Robert Swanson. Swanson was aspiring to make a stronghold in the VC industry and encouraged Dr. Boyer's idea. He along with a few other venture capitalists invested in the company as an act of speculation. To quote a venture capitalist who invested in the company about the level of risk they took on, "Very high. I figured better than 50–50 we'd lose it. But it's rare when the odds on a new technology are better than 50 percent." Second thoughts? "Not at all. If it worked, the rewards would be obvious" (Hughes, 2011, p. 41).

This speculative act of investment evolved later. While in the case of Genentech what we get to see is wild speculation, with time, the social practices of financial valuation of DBFs evolved in such a way that it is both 'speculative' and at the same time real. This is not to say that speculation is a specific feature of financialised innovations, but rather that the speculation here is much more complex than the simple non-financialised[7] investments and thereby constituting its own reality in congruence with the level of complexity. The complexity only further increases depending on the nature of innovations, and typically biological mechanisms are highly complex and therefore the higher the level of speculation.

In a non-financialised production process, the logic of risk versus returns operates in a single circuit where returns are determined by speculating on the demand side. In this scenario, the level of risk is only determined by the demand-side factors. If the final consumer demand meets the expectation of the investment, then the venture turns profitable. But in the context of MBT innovations under the financialisation logic, that is not the case. Here speculation is much more complex and operates at multiple levels. Financial actors typically invest in an innovative idea that is supposedly novel expecting a market disruption. This investment in the novel innovative idea is a supply-side event which may or may not manifest as anticipated. Hence, under financialised innovations, the first level of risk is in the supply-side process. Therefore, given this element of risk, financial investments in these ventures come in rounds conditional upon certain milestones that the firm reaches. One of the instruments that provide real-time assurance to investors in this process is the patent. But in the case of drug development, coming up with a novel innovation and patenting it is only one part of the story. For the innovation to reach its end user, it has to go through a cumbersome clinical trial process which is a heavy investment and highly risky affair. As mentioned previously, only one in every five drugs that enter clinical trials turns out successful. Therefore, the investors encourage these innovators to either out-licence their innovations, offer an IPO, or undergo an M&A so that they can get an exit with returns on their investment. The present value of these innovations or the firm is determined through a valuation process based on the potential future earnings. This process entails an active construction of markets by the financial actors. It is based on this valuation that transactions take place between a pharmaceutical firm and DBF. For the pharmaceutical industry, which is in dire need of innovation, the patent portfolios of these firms help it make safe bets. However, even the pharmaceutical industry risks itself by investing in these innovations since there is no guarantee that an early stage innovation would be necessarily successful in the clinical trial process, as well as in terms of demand. But, since all of these innovations are monopolistic, the returns that these innovations ensure in case of success are obvious. With every milestone, while the venture capitalists try to reduce their risk and make returns, the pharmaceutical industry, conversely, entertains a certain amount of risk speculating on the prospective returns that may come out of the innovative activity of the DBFs. This is the new market game that the MBT industry has ushered in—a highly speculative and complex market space mediated by the dynamic of multiple levels of risk vs returns.

MBT—The Real and the Speculation

As mentioned in the previous section, the scientific advancements that gave birth to MBT in the late 1970s in the US coincided with the neoliberal promotion of supply-side economics. The subsequent legislation and the rulings on patenting are clearly significant factors in the growth of this industry. Globally, the advancement of MBT led to a post-Fordist setup of pharmaceutical R&D (Lehman, 2010). Starting from the 1930s till the emergence of MBT, which is considered as the golden age of medicinal chemistry, pharmaceutical production used to largely take place in vertically integrated firms. However, with the rise of MBT, there was an emergence of new relationships between the big pharmaceutical companies and DBFs in the form of licencing deals and M&As. Between 1997 and 2002, the five largest pharmaceutical companies in-licenced six to ten products from DBFs and earned 28%–80% of their revenue (Demain, 2010). The progress of the MBT industry that took place during this time is exemplified by the fact that it had just two drug/vaccine approvals in 1982, none in 1983/1984, one in 1985, and went up to 32 in 2000 (Demain, 2010). The number of patents granted to DBFs also rose from 1,500 in 1985 to 9,000 in 1999 (Demain, 2010).

However, 30 years after the establishment of the first DBF, a study by Pisano (2006) noted that the promise of MBT that there would be a revolution in drug development and generation of vast profits is not yet fulfilled. Except for a few firms such as Genentech and Amgen, most firms did not report profits. Similarly, Nightingale and Martin (2004) characterise the biotech revolution as a myth based on empirical evidence proving that the outputs of biotech R&D failed to keep pace with the increased funding. In their study, it is shown that as one moves along the innovation path work from "basic research to target discovery, target validation and into clinical development, evidence for a biotechnology revolution rapidly diminishes" (Nightingale & Martin, 2004, p. 564). Using time-series data between 1989 and 2003 and indicators such as the number of publications in the area of genomics, patents of therapeutically active compounds in USPTO and World Patent Index, business expenditure on pharmaceutical R&D and Food and Drug Administration (FDA) approval of prescriptive drugs, the study concludes that the promises made by MBT have mostly remained a myth. In fact, Lehman's (2010) research also proves the same point that MBT industry in the US, instead of proving itself as a revolutionary technology, has become a part of the conventional blockbuster drug business model.

After the global financial crisis in 2008, almost a third of publicly listed DBFs went bust by 2011 in the UK (Birch, 2017). A similar trend was witnessed across the globe. Table 0.3 provides details about the number and amount of VC funds and IPO over the years across the globe.

The data from Table 0.3 indicates a steep decline in the number of IPOs during 2008, which increased only gradually till 2013. However, it can be witnessed how by 2014, the market capitalisation soared in terms of the number of IPO deals. In 2014, the total market capitalisation of the global biotech industry crossed one trillion USD (Birch, 2017). But what is interesting is that such increasing levels of market capitalisation were not due to any substantial increase in either products or services by these firms in the market (Birch, 2017). Even in 2014, the DBFs were producing very disproportionately similar to what Pisano observed in 2006. Birch (2017) attributes this to the rent deriving nature of the assets such as patents of the firms and the role of speculation in the biotech market that was described in the previous section behind this increasing capitalisation. What this then suggests is that, the global speculative markets particularly in the MBT sector are perpetually in a state of risk/potential "crisis" and the implications of such crisis being that MBT firms increasingly turning as Ponzi schemes (Mirowski, 2012).

Table 0.3 Global VC and IPO Deals Over Time

S. No	Year	IPO		VC	
		No of Deals	Amount Raised per Deal (Avg.) Million USD	No of Deals	Amount Raised (Avg.) Million USD
1.	2005	45	41	NA	NA
2.	2006	49	41	336	5,589
3.	2007	51	58	386	5,547
4.	2008	6	22	358	4,623
5.	2009	10	92.8	315	3,771
6.	2010	19	51	324	3,557
7.	2011	13	81.4	292	3,824
8.	2012	17	53.6	281	3,925
9.	2013	43	72.5	322	4,539
10.	2014	90	72.3	341	5,879
11.	2015	65	81.5	387	10,126
12.	2016	49	58	344	8,483
13.	2017	55	98.4	333	8,768

Source: As cited in Morrison and Lähteenmäki (2017); Huggett (2018)
NA—Not Available

Political and Legal Changes That Led to the Constitution of the MBT Ecosystem in the US

Whether it is about the VC supporting the emergence of an industry or universities aggressively commercialising their research or patents acting as assets, all of them are in one way also a result of the deliberate political and legal changes that took place in the US in the late '70s and early '80s "to benefit the biotech industry and thereby construct a specific technological market" (Birch, 2006, p. 95). This section provides an overview of several such measures by the state in the US that reflect upon the neoliberal nature of the state in the US. Melinda Copper (2008) through her study argues that from President Ronald Reagan's neoliberal era, broad political changes took place in general to support the supply-side of the economy and specifically more so in the MBT sector. Firstly, the birth of the biotech business model coincided with the relaxation of liabilities associated with VC in the late '70s when the Department of Labour in the US legalised investment of pension funds into venture funds, which was treated as illegal earlier (Roth, 2000). Also, the special provisions on capital gains tax which ended in the year 1969 were renewed again in the year 1978 (Roth, 2000). This led to an increased investment in VC funds (VCFs), which were investing in innovative enterprises such as MBT. Another crucial impetus towards the growth of the MBT industry in the US is the dramatic increase in federal funding for life science research standing next to heavily funded defence and obligating universities to increasingly perform research for commercial interests (Cooper, 2008). Prior to this, in 1980, two important regulations were enacted. The first is the Bayh-Dole Act, which allowed universities to hold patent rights for federally funded research and eliminated restrictions for their licencing. This provision was later extended in 1983 to small and medium enterprises as well that received federal funding. In the same year, the enactment of the Stevenson-Wylder Technology Transfer Act enabled the creation of a TTO at NIH to transfer the publicly funded research outputs to the industry. At least 15 significant regulations were enacted during the 1980s that benefitted the private biotech sector in the US.[8] The ruling in the *Diamond vs. Chakrabarty* patenting case, which ruled that genetically modified bacteria are patentable in and of themselves apart from their use in the research process, also played a significant role. This led to the opening of the window for patenting of cell lines, DNA, genes, animals, and any other living organisms that were "sufficiently" modified (Krimsky, 2003). Along with these, many other incentives such as the 1981 Economic Recovery Tax Act, which awarded tax credits for R&D; the 1984 Patent Term Restoration Act; and the 1987 Presidential Executive Order for pushing more technology transfer from federally funded universities played a key role in the ascent and progress of this industry (Loeppky, 2005). Finally, the missing regulations of drug price control in the US also played a crucial role in the proliferation of the medical technology industry in the US that helped in upholding the big pharma monopolies (Lehman, 2010). All of these measures indicate the deliberate role of the state in the proliferation of the private biotechnology industry in the US.

What Does This Book Attempt to Do?

In the previous sections, we have seen how neoliberal policymaking has determined the entanglement of the "bio"+ "economic" in the US context- and the role of state, academia, and finance capital in this process. The earlier discussion also suggests how MBT innovations are largely taking place under a new accumulation regime dominated by finance capital. In this process, the role of the state is relegated to becoming an active agent of private capital accumulation by intervening in markets in contrast to what is propounded by the theory of neoliberalism. The enactment of patent laws and legislations that allowed publicly funded research to be commercialised has provided a new impetus to academic institutions to monopolise knowledge, distancing it from the social realm where knowledge is considered a common property. This monopolisation of knowledge has in turn led to monopolistic technologies that started appropriating a common pool of resources for private profits. Nevertheless, the Indian story of this entanglement process is an important gap that needs to be addressed not least because of the implications it has for various social actors. In India, the neoliberal reforms were gradually introduced during the mid-1980s, and with the balance of payment crisis, the

Indian state liberalised its markets in 1991 and deregulated a vast majority of sectors free from state intervention. Coincidentally, the emergence of biotech phenomenon in India also took place during the same period. Therefore, the development of the Indian biotech sector right from its emergence took place under a political-economic system that implicates a variety of social actors and institutions with consequences for large sections of society.

Also, if one looks at the developments in the biotech industry, the period after 1995 witnessed a growth in industrial activity with the emergence of DBFs and large pharmaceutical companies diversifying their businesses into biotech. This is because of the change in the intellectual property rights (IPR) regime in the country after India became a signatory of the World Trade Organization's Trade-Related Intellectual Property Rights Agreement (TRIPS). After this harmonisation of patent laws, subsidiaries of transnational firms like Eli Lilly and Glaxo Smith Kline also entered into the biotech arena in India (Arora, 2005). The biotech industry in India developed in clusters such as Bangalore, Hyderabad, Pune, Delhi NCR, and Gujarat (FICCI, 2015) consisting of biopharma, bioagri, bioindustrial, and bioservices sub-sectors. The industry was valued at 51 billion USD in 2018 and is expected to reach 100 billion USD by 2025 (DIPP & DBT, 2017). Biopharma is the leading sub-sector contributing up to 55% of the value in 2018. Today, India is among the top-12 biotech destinations in the world and the third in Asia-Pacific (Frost & Sullivan, 2016). In the past, India did not have many start-ups due to the absence of an innovative ecosystem, low R&D by the private sector, absence of translation research centres, lack of VC, and lack of incubator facilities and infrastructure (Saberwal, 2016; Ramani & Maria, 2005). Currently, there are 2,689 biotech start-ups and more than 600 full-fledged biotech firms in India (BIRAC[a], 2019, *BioSpectrum*, 2019). The Government of India (GoI) aims to increase the number of start-ups to 10,000 by 2024 (DBT, 2019a). Table 0.4 provides an overview of the sectoral composition of biotech start-ups.

While all of these developments and numbers indicate an upward trajectory of biotech in India, what went behind these developments is a story that this book engages with. The book is interested in examining the conditions under which the biotech phenomenon emerged in India; the role of various actors and institutions, particularly the state, academia, and finance

Table 0.4 Composition of Biotech Start-Ups

S. No	Biotech Sector	Percentage of Start-Ups
1.	Biopharma	57
2.	Bioagri	10
3.	Bioindustrial	9
4.	Bio-IT/CRO*/research	24

Source: ABLE (n.d.)
* Contract research Organisation

capital in these developments; and the implications they have on the social role of the institutions.

Approach, Methods, and Data Sources

The study undertakes a critical political economy approach to analyse the developments in India's MBT sector. I argue in the book that the evolutionary trajectory of MBT in India depicts a picture that prioritises private capital accumulation at the cost of public resources. This is antithetical to the theory of neoliberalism, which postulates that markets are *in and of themselves efficient*. I unfold my argument over the next four chapters by examining the role of various actors and institutions, particularly the state, academia, and finance capital and their role in the process of capital accumulation through MBT start-ups. For this purpose, different forms of data sources, including both primary and secondary, were deployed. Semi-structured in-depth interviews with academic scientists, policymakers, MBT start-up founders and their employees, and university TTO employees were conducted. A wide range of secondary data sources, including various reports published by government organisations such as Department of Biotechnology (DBT), Council for Scientific and Industrial Research (CSIR), Biotechnology Industry Research Assistance Council (BIRAC), Department of Science and Technology, Comptroller and Auditor General (CAG) of India, policy documents from GoI institutions, websites of MBT firms and academic institutions, Indian Patent Office website, business magazines, reports of various consultancy firms, and newspaper articles were used.

In the following chapter, I begin by examining the origins of MBT both as an epistemological and commercial endeavour in India. I show how the state's role in the development of the biotech sector is guided solely by the prospects of economic growth and private capital accumulation, even at the cost of the larger public good. This early history of biotech developments in the country is traced using archival material from various sources, including public organisations, such as the DBT, newspaper reports, websites of academic institutions, and commercial MBT firms, as well as other relevant literature. Further, by employing the case study method, seven first-of-their-kind successful MBT commercial initiatives in India in the public sector, PPPs, and private sector were examined. These case studies illustrate in detail the neoliberal nature of the Indian state and the complex networks of accumulation of first-generation MBT firms in India. I show how public-sector units were subjected to negligence by the Indian state and were made part of the global value chain of vaccine markets catering to the interests of multinational pharmaceutical firms, leaving behind the larger public good of achieving self-sufficiency in vaccine production. The cases of PPPs illustrate how public resources were appropriated by private capital, negating the propaganda that PPPs are essentially risk-sharing agreements by both public and private partners. Further, the case studies of successful first-generation private firms show the significant role of the state in their accumulation process. However, much of the success of these first-generation firms took place before an organised ecosystem for MBT innovations in the country started coming up.

It was in the year 2007, a watershed moment in the history of biotechnology in the country, an organised ecosystem in the name of National Biotechnology Development Strategy came up with the state acting as the central agent, ensuring all the elements of the ecosystem. Broader structural changes such as deregulation of financial markets, liberalising foreign VC investments, took place a little before this in the year 2005. With the help of in-depth interviews from policymakers and other relevant information from various secondary sources, in Chapter 2, I discuss the central role of the state in the ecosystem in terms of budgetary sanctions, infrastructure support, institutional support, and favourable policy environment.

Thereafter, using secondary data from the Securities and Exchange Board of India (SEBI), business consultancy firms, and policy documents, in Chapter 3, I examine the role of financial actors and institutions, particularly in terms of VC investments in the MBT sector. I argue in this chapter that while there is an overall increasing trend of VC investments across sectors over time, the share of MBT is limited. However, I further argue that these increasing trends of investment are going to reflect in the MBT sector, as well give various kinds of incentives provided by the Indian state both for financial actors and MBT start-ups.

In Chapter 4, I examine the role of academia and academic scientists. This chapter is based on in-depth interviews with academic scientists and TTO employees in addition to the use of secondary data from different sources on the number of patents filed and granted to some of the leading academic institutes in the country. Information was also sought under the Right to Information Act from DBT autonomous institutions to understand the extent of commercialisation these institutions were undergoing. In this chapter, I argue that, while the academia-industry interaction existed in India's academic institutions right from Independence, the nature of these interactions changed over time with the global harmonisation of patent laws and the rising prominence of the knowledge economy. Further, in this chapter, I deconstruct the neoliberal myth of incentivising the supply-side by showing the disproportionate ratio between the number of patents filed and granted to the academic institutions. What appears from this empirical data is that Indian academic institutions are turning into patent factories. While the frenzy of patenting in Indian academic institutions could not deliver the promised results, it caused a loss to the public exchequer.

After examining the role of key actors in the MBT ecosystem, in Chapter 5, I examine the process of production and accumulation in MBT start-ups. Based on in-depth interviews with start-up founders (20) and employees (14), I show how the production process differs in these firms from those of highly established firms. Examining the exit strategies of these start-ups, I argue based on Marx's idea of capital accumulation (M-C-M') that the so-called successful start-ups enable what is called a *double-layered accumulation* in a single production process. I further argue that this is a specific phenomenon of knowledge-based enterprises that thrive on monopolistic technologies. Following this empirical discussion that is elaborated on in over four chapters, the final chapter of the book presents its conclusion, arguing that if it were not for the neoliberal Indian state, MBT would not have existed in the country in the form it currently does.

Notes

1 The sequencing of human genome through the most celebrated HGP was to come up with a sequence of 'normal/ desirable' organisations of human life at the molecular level.

2 Basic science research is conducted to answer fundamental questions but not with any immediate social or economically relevant applications in mind. On the other hand, applied research is carried out with the objective of coming out with applications of such research in real time.

3 rDNA is a technology that uses enzymes to cut and paste together DNA sequences of interest. The recombined DNA sequences can be placed into vehicles called vectors that ferry the DNA into a suitable host cell where it can be copied or expressed.

4 For a more detailed description of how patenting phenomenon of basic science research began, please refer to Hughes (2001) who presents these details through oral histories from the discoverers of rDNA technology and Neils Reimer, the TTO officer at the Stanford.

5 It is no exaggeration to say that this is currently the order of the day, particularly with regard to the MBT ecosystem.

6 Pharmacogenomics is a technique used to rationalise the clinical trial process by classifying the trail subjects based on their genetic response to drugs.

7 Financialisation refers to circulation of capital as an end in itself for generation of surplus value rather than investing in commodity production.

8 For a brief discussion on these regulations, please refer to Birch (2006).

Chapter 1

The Beginnings

In India, the introduction of neoliberal reforms started in the 1980s (Kohli, 2006), and gradually, by 1991, with complete liberalisation of markets—except for a few strategic sectors—there was a transformation of India's political and economic spheres. With neoliberalism as a guiding principle, the state was offering large-scale incentives for private capital accumulation, weakening the public-sector units (PSU) and encouraging public-private partnerships (PPP). It was during the same period that biotechnology was also rising to prominence in India primarily because of the potential it has to offer for economic growth. As a result, what was witnessed is that, right from the beginning, the biotechnology trajectory was predicated on neoliberal economic principles, and the growth objective was formulated in such a way that it caters to the interests of a few while leaving behind the many. This chapter, by unearthing the policies, processes, and strategies, explains how the biotechnology paradigm in India, right from the beginning, was set in process by the state and its institutions with the objective of enabling the expansion of private capital using public resources.

One of the major transformations that took place with the neoliberal restructuring is the decline and reconfiguration of the PSUs. Also, with economic liberalisation, the state actively encouraged business models like the PPPs and encouraged capital accumulation by providing various incentives to the private industry. The consequence of such intervention is a higher public cost for narrow private benefits. This phenomenon is witnessed in the Indian biotech sector right from its emergence due to its convergence with the onset of neoliberalism in the country. In order to demonstrate this, case studies of seven first-generation commercial MBT endeavours consisting of one PSU, two PPPs, and four in the private sector that are first-of-their-kind initiatives in the country are discussed in this chapter. The PSU discussed is that of Bharat Immunological and Biological Corporation Limited (BIBICOL) established by the Department of Biotechnology (DBT) in 1989, which subsequently underwent several changes in its structure and business model during the period of economic reforms. This is also the first PSU established by the DBT for vaccine manufacturing to make India self-sufficient in vaccine production.

DOI: 10.4324/9781003292104-2

The PPP projects include the Genomed project, which was a partnership between the Institute for Genomics and Integrative Biology (IGIB) and Nicolas Primal India Limited (NPIL) established in 2002 and The Centre for Genomic Applications (TCGA), a partnership between IGIB and the Chatterjee Management Services (CMS) established in the year 2003. Genomed is a first-of-its-kind knowledge equity venture with a public-sector institution and private industry and TCGA is an establishment of necessary infrastructure and resources for enhancing biotechnology research in the country. Thereafter, case studies of four private biotech enterprises in the country that were established during the early stage of the biotech scenario and are first-of-their-kind initiatives are discussed. These firms include Biocon, Astra Research Centre India (ARCI), Shanta Biotechnics, and Strand Life Sciences (SLiSc). These case study firms illustrate the role of the state and the network of actors involved in the capital accumulation process during the emergent moment of the biotech scenario in the country.

The Beginnings of the Biotech Scenario in India

The initial impetus towards the growth of the biotech sector in India came from the state. This is exemplified by the fact that till the 1990s, there was no active involvement of the private sector in biotechnology-related activities, except for a handful of firms. A few subsidiaries of multinational firms, along with a few Indian firms with borrowed technologies from the West, were engaging in biotech activities (Kumar, 1987). As such, the initial policy engagement with biotechnology took place in India for the first time during the sixth five-year plan, which led to the establishment of the National Biotechnology Board (NBTB) under the then prime minister (PM) Indira Gandhi in the year 1982 (Chaturvedi, 2007). Around the same time in 1984, the International Union for Pure and Applied Chemistry's (IUPAC) seventh International Biotechnology Symposium was held in New Delhi, the first time in any developing country (Ghose & Bisaria, 2000). And in 1986, the United Nations Industrial Development Organization established a component of the International Centre for Genetic Engineering and Biotechnology in New Delhi (Fan & Watanabe, 2008). The Government of India (GoI) since the 1990s has supported this sector in a large way through various incentives such as tax exemption, providing of venture capital (VC), and price control exemptions on the export of healthcare products, to list a major few (Gulifeiya & Aljunid, 2012). Before this recognition by the Indian state, microbiology even as an academic endeavour wasn't so prominent in India. During the 1950s and '60s, only a few research institutes were engaging in microbiology research, including the Indian Institute of Science (IISc), Bangalore; National Chemical Laboratory (NCL), Pune; and the Department of Applied Chemistry of University of Calcutta (Bhargava & Chakrabarti, 1991). It was only in 1977 that India witnessed the emergence of a full-fledged research centre entirely dedicated to research in microbiology in the form of the Centre for Cellular and Molecular Biology (CCMB) established by the Council for Scientific and Industrial Research (CSIR) with Prof. Pushpa M Bhargava as its first director (Singh, 2016). Interestingly, this was the same year that the discovery of rDNA technology took place, which later paved the way for the commercial proliferation of the biotechnology industry. Bhargava, who returned to India after working at the University of Wisconsin and National Institute of Medical Research, UK, was a strong proponent of India's participation in the molecular biology-based scientific paradigm. He is also one of the major reasons behind the establishment of NBTB, along with the initiative of the Indian National Science Academy, CSIR, and DST (Bhargava, 2009). However, Bhargava writing in an article in *Current Science*, mentions that he was not happy with the establishment of NBTB. For one, what he was wishing for was a dedicated board of biotechnology that engaged in three activities—namely, research, development, and production. Secondly, though NBTB had an executive secretary, the real powers rested with the secretary of DST, and it also had very little funds. He along with a few other scientists at that time wrote to Rajiv Gandhi, then PM of India, expressing their discontent with NBTB and requested a dedicated DBT (Bhargava & Chakrabarti, 1991). Thereafter, in 1986, the DBT as an autonomous department was established with Dr. S Rama Chandran, someone who comes from an industrial background, as its first member secretary (Vijay Raghavan, 2016). Also, a Product and Industry Development (PID) division was started in DBT in 1989 to transfer the research results of government-funded institutionally developed technologies to the industry (Ghosh, 1996). India was the first country across the globe to have a separate department for biotechnology (DBT, n.d.-b). Ramachandran says, with regard to such generous sanction by the state, "Prime Minister Rajiv Gandhi recognised the pace at which biological sciences were growing globally that 'unless we leap forward, there is a no way of catching up with rest of the world'" (ibid.). The main reason pointed out for taking the initiative in such a big way was articulated by DBT as "because many of our macro-economic issues of growth were *subsumed* (emphasis original) within that science's development" (ibid.). Established with such enthusiasm, the department received sharp criticism from inside about its underperformance than expected with respect to its industrial activity. Bhargava, who was a member of its high-powered Scientific Advisory Committee (SAC), voiced a relentless criticism about the functioning of this institution for over a decade. In an article in *Current Science* (1991, p. 516) in response to the question, "What would have been the scenario if DBT had not been there?" he replied with "Not very different from what it is today." Writing in another article in the *Economic and Political Weekly* (1995) assessing the DBT's performance, he said,

> Whatever has happened in the area of biotechnology in the country has been outside of the purview or influence of the DBT and would have

happened even if the DBT was not there. In the eyes of the industry, including the fledgling biotechnology industry in the country, and the people of the country, the DBT has been a non-entity.

(Bhargava, 1995, p. 3050)

He also expressed that such lethargy with which DBT worked towards industrial co-operation would lead to 'neo-colonialism'[1] and appealed to the government to take risks on behalf of the private sector, as he opines that the *latter* would not take risks in a country like ours (Bhargava & Chakrabarti, 1991). The basis for Bhargava's criticism of DBT is that it has not performed as expected with respect to support of industrial activity in India. However, Ramachandran, the first secretary of DBT, negates this by saying that the initial focus of DBT had been in the development of capabilities and setting up of institutions (Ramachandran, 1991b). It was only a matter of time before the DBT involved itself in the activities that Bhargava was suggesting. As mentioned previously, DBT started a PID in 1989 itself, and in its 2005 draft document of National Biotechnology Development Strategy–I (NBDS-I), it encouraged PPP, recommending an allocation of 30% of its budget towards PPP activities (Jayaraman, 2005). NBDS-I, in order to develop human resources, also recommended a PPP model of PhDs named Bio-Edu-Grid, which is a network of universities and industries to facilitate the pooling of resources (DBT, 2005). This private-industry-friendly activity in the biotech sector in India coincided with the transformation of the macroeconomic policy of India into a more market-friendly one. The Science & Technology (S&T) plan during the eighth plan period calls for the aligning of S&T with the New Industrial Policy of 1991 (Planning Commission, 1992) that was championing the cause of private industry and foreign investments (Patnaik, 2016). This neoliberal transformation of the economy in turn shaped the development of the Indian biotech sector right from its emergence.

In 1990, to institutionalise the commercial linkages of academia with industry, a new entity named Biotechnology Industry Consortium Limited (BCIL) was established (Ramachandran, 1991b). The company was promoted by DBT, and its core capital of Rs. 53.7 million was provided by financial institutions, including the Industrial Development Bank of India (IDBI), Industrial Credit and Investment Corporation of India (ICICI), Industrial Finance Corporation of India (IFCI), Unit Trust of India (UTI), and contributions from the corporate sector, including Ranbaxy Pvt Ltd, Cadila Laboratories Pvt Ltd and Glaxo India Pvt Ltd (Kharbanda, 2004). Further, recently, in 2012, it established another institution—namely, Biotechnology Industry Research Assistance Council (BIRAC)—specifically to encourage PPPs and help start commercial establishments by providing capital at various stages of development. Currently, the introduction page of the newly revamped DBT website ends by saying, "The future is bright with DBT collaborating with industry in new programmes. We welcome all stakeholders to join this historical march forward!" (DBT, n.d.-b).

This evolutionary trajectory of the biotech sector in India shows that economic considerations, more specifically the goal of economic growth through the promotion of private industries, assumed the central objective of the biotech strategy of India. One can witness a clear co-production of the economy and technoscience and the development priorities of the government here. In the following section, the case of BIBICOL, the only PSU established by the DBT which is still functioning, is critically examined to explicate how it ended up serving the interests of private capital.

From Producer of Vaccines to Supplier in the Global Value Chain: Trajectories of BIBICOL

Though India has an early history of institutionalisation of vaccine production right from the colonial period, actual vaccine production in India was started by the DBT (Madhavi, 2007). India as a part of the World Health Organization's (WHO) Alma Alta Declaration of "Health for All" introduced an Expanded Programme of Immunisation in 1978, and further intensified these efforts through the Universal Immunisation Programme in 1985 and National Technology Mission on Immunization in 1986 (ibid.). DBT was also established as a separate DBT in 1986. As part of such intensified efforts, the Ministry of Health and Family Welfare and DBT were given responsibility for the successful implementation of the immunisation project with a clear mandate to make India self-sufficient in vaccine production (Ramachandran, 1991b). DBT established two PSUs—namely, BIBICOL and Indian Vaccine Company Limited (IVCOL)—for this purpose. IVCOL was incorporated as a joint venture unit between DBT, Indian Petrochemicals Corporation Limited (IPCL), and Pasteur and Merieux Serum and Vaccines (PMSV) a PSU in France. The idea behind this partnership was that PMSV would transfer the technology required to IVCOL and IVCOL would manufacture the vaccines. IVCOL was put to a halt in 1992 because PMSV turned into a private company, and since Indian markets were liberalised by 1992, PMSV refused to transfer the technology (Madhavi, 2005). IVCOL now is non-functional, leaving BIBICOL as the only PSU established by DBT that is still functioning after being declared as a sick unit in 2000 (Madhavi, 2007). This makes BIBICOL an interesting case to pursue.

The initial capital required for the project was provided by DBT, along with several other financial institutions (Somasekhar, 2000). The main focus of BIBICOL was on formulating the oral polio vaccine (OPV) through a technology transfer agreement called "Technology Consultancy Co-Operation" with a Russian firm named Institute of Poliomyelitis and Viral Encephalitis (IPVE; Madhavi, 2007). IPVE, in exchange, promised to provide the basic know-how on the condition that India would bulk import OPV during the first phase of the agreement. This relationship of BIBICOL with IPVE formed a part of the bilateral agreement between India and Russia for long-term scientific co-operation in 1987 (Planning Commission, 1992). Within five years after its establishment, i.e. in 1994, BIBICOL went for an initial public offering (IPO) and was listed in the Bombay, Kolkata, and Delhi stock exchanges to raise the capital (BIBICOL, n.d.). By then, the global biotech scenario, especially in the US that began much earlier than in India, was entwined with the financial markets. In the Indian case, however, even today, there are hardly any biotech companies that are publicly traded. Biocon, the first private biotech firm in India established in 1977, went for an IPO only in 2004.

The story of BIBICOL has several interesting turns. Pasteur Institute of India (PII) had set up a unit for the production of OPV before BIBICOL (in 1969) with support from WHO and GoI. The vaccine technology was also imported from IPVE and the seed virus that was necessary was procured by Dr. A. B. Sabin, who originally developed OPV (Ramachandran, 2008). PII had successfully produced six batches of the vaccine and had to stop production after its seventh batch was allegedly found to be virulent (ibid.). Madhavi (2007) argues, after this incident, for nearly two decades, there were no efforts by the state to reinitiate the production after taking any corrective measures; conversely, it depended on imports deviating from the initial mandate of encouraging indigenous production. BIBICOL was the next serious initiative in the public sector for fostering indigenous production. However, BIBICOL was also not successful in developing vaccines domestically due to various reasons. The most important reason was the termination of BIBICOL's contract with IPVE, subsequent to the objection of the United Nations Children's Fund (UNICEF) since IPVE did not have the Good Manufacturing Practices certification mandated by WHO for the procurement of vaccines (ibid.). UNICEF was one of the major buyers from BIBICOL, and due to the issues with certification, BIBICOL was forced to terminate the contract with IPVE (ibid.). It should be noted that, as per the agreement between BIBICOL and IPVE, the technical know-how of vaccine production was supposed to be transferred to BIBICOL after importing six batches of vaccine. This premature termination of the contract deprived BIBICOL of acquiring the vaccine production technology, and the firm ended up importing vaccines from multinational companies (MNCs) like SmithKline Belgium and BioPharma, US, rather than manufacturing vaccines by itself (ibid.).

Besides, vaccine development turned out to be financially unviable for BIBICOL in post-liberalised India due to market competition. Of the total 900 million doses of vaccine required for India, private firms were supplying nearly 620 million (Somasekhar, 2000). BIBICOL's share in vaccine supply came down with their presence, and, subsequently, it recorded substantial losses in revenue. Consequently, in the year 2000, the company was declared as a sick unit by the GoI and was handed over to the Board for Financial and Industrial Reconstruction (BIFR) to restructure its business and diversify production completely based on imports (Mishra, 2001).

What emerges from the case of BIBICOL is that while DBT is mandated with building national capabilities for self-sufficiency, BIBICOL ended up as an importer of vaccines. Also, the case of BIBICOL depicts how PSUs are weakened with the implementation of neoliberal principles even if it leads to pushing back some of the most important social priorities. The restructuring of BIBICOL by BIFR is a part of common practice by the Indian state to weaken PSUs either by restructuring their business models or by entirely disinvesting as a part of its neoliberal commitment. In this process, the entire purpose for which BIBICOL was established was side-lined and its initial mandate of making the country self-sufficient in vaccine production never took fruition.

With the restructuring of BIBICOL, which is well equipped with infrastructure and resources, it became an agent to outsource (obligatory import) for MNCs to bring their goods to the market. In fact, scholars have argued that the MNCs, in nexus with international organisations such as the WHO, take control of the markets in developing countries (Puliyel & Madhavi, 2008; Baru, 2003; Madhavi, 2007; Madhavi, 2013,) and the case of BIBICOL also depicts a similar scenario. The strategy here appears to be very similar albeit in a different form that the global economy witnessed in the form of international value chains (IVCs) to outsource work for cost-cutting in the production process and accumulate the ensuring surplus. The only difference is, in the case of IVCs, higher value is captured through cost-cutting by outsourcing work to resource-poor countries and in the case where obligatory import strategies are implemented, higher value is captured through market expansion.

What is also interesting in the case of BIBICOL is, while in the popular imagination it is only private firms and institutions that act as agents for outsourced work, BIBICOL's case shows how PSUs also get to partner in the global accumulation strategy. After restructuring, BIBICOL ventured in a big way by depending completely on the imports and brought final goods of MNCs to the market. The original mandate with which BIBICOL was established was never accomplished. From the case of BIBICOL, it can be witnessed how initiatives from the state could end up serving the interests of the private industry while at the same time forgoing the larger interests of its people. In the following section, we discuss how the PPP-based initiatives in the biotech sector also ended up in a similar fashion.

Trajectories of the PPP Models in Biotechnology

While the public-sector biotech firm in India has become part of the networks of accumulation deviating from their initial mandate of serving the larger national interest, the PPPs, which were aggressively promoted by the state as part of the economic reforms, have also ended up in a similar process. The only difference is, while in the case of BIBICOL it is MNCs that have benefitted, in our cases of PPP, it is the firms of Indian origin that benefitted from public resources. The stated objective behind PPPs, vigorously advocated by the World Bank is that it provides a *win-win situation* for both the private investor and public at large within a given time period.

However, the winner can always be a single party if the power relations between the parties are not balanced. The PPPs in India's biotech sector bear clear testimony to this. I elaborate on this argument by drawing from two PPPs in the biotechnology sector that were established during the early days of the biotech scenario in the country.

Appropriation of Public in PPP Models: The Cases of Genomed and TCGA

The two PPPs that will be discussed here are Genomed and TCGA. Genomed is a PPP between IGIB and NPIL established in the year 2002.[2] It is a 50:50 joint venture between IGIB, a publicly funded research institution, and a corporate entity NPIL (Rediff, 2000). The investment promised by NPIL in the project was around Rs 1,000 million over a period of ten years (Ramachandran, 2000). The PPP is formed based on the principle that IGIB will conduct research and develop technologies, and NPIL would use them in their production process. Genomed also has another laboratory space at Well Quest, which is a clinical research organisation located in the Well Spring Hospital set up by NPIL that conducts clinical trials for big pharmaceutical companies. The association of Genomed with Well Quest was a well-thought-out strategy for two reasons. First is, given the application of pharmacogenomics[3] in the clinical trial process, the location of Genomed at this space is one that is based on economic contributions that it could generate to the NPIL (Sunder Rajan, 2005). Second, by virtue of the location of Genomed at the Well Spring Hospital, there is a seamless supply of biological material (disease information, health records, etc.) that can be converted into valuable information and thereby potential applications.

Genomed is a first-of-its-kind venture in India. The idea behind this partnership, according to the Principal Scientific Advisor, GoI, is that "knowledge is the commodity and it has been equated like 'equity'" (Principal Scientific Advisor, n.d.), and IGIB terms this relationship as a "knowledge alliance" (IGIB, n.d.-a). This alliance is formed in such a way that the areas of co-operation for which it is agreed upon are to be exclusive, implying that in the areas agreed upon, IGIB's research is conducted exclusively for NPIL. All the technologies that come out of IGIB's research, while they are jointly patented, IGIB is obligated to licence them only to NPIL (Business Line, 2000). This PPP venture is claimed as a milestone in Indian genomics history (CSIR, n.d.).

However, what is important to understand from this arrangement is who gets to benefit from this set-up and at what cost? In order to address this question, it is important to understand "where value resides as biology becomes an information science, and what work and whose agencies are required to create these values?" Sunder Rajan (2006, p. 41) posed this in his celebrated work *Biocapital*. He explains that in order to find answers to these questions, it is important to understand the "circulation of information and changing forms of corporate activity" (Sunder Rajan, 2006, p. 41). In the case of Genomed, as already explained, the circulation of information, which emanates from the processing of biological materials, is from IGIB to NPIL. IGIB associates with hospitals such as Well Spring, National Institute of Mental Health and Neuro Sciences, and All India Institute of Medical Sciences (Ramachandran, 2000; AIIMS, 2005) for biological material and researches on them using public resources to obtain information which is valuable. The 'valuable' information thus obtained is used by the corporate entity NPIL for its business purposes. In this process of circulation, the agency and actors involved are the scientists at IGIB, the publicly funded IGIB as an institution, and NPIL, who get exclusive rights on this research and also on the products that may subsequently be developed. What is also interesting to note from this particular PPP is that while patents in a way provide a monopoly over the research results, in this 'knowledge partnership,' one gets to witness the prevention of even the research activity by IGIB in the areas agreed upon to any other entities. A former director of IGIB—under whose leadership this initiative took place—in an interview was quoted saying, "[T]the domains [of research] that have been mentioned [in the PPP agreement] will be exclusive to NPIL" (as cited in Business Line, 2000). What one gets to understand from this collaboration is that while the public-sector institutions are to conduct research and generate valuable information using public resources, this valuable information should only be put to use for the benefit of the private partner. In this process, what is forgone is the long-cherished principle of autonomy of publicly funded research institutions where IGIB is restricted to perform research in areas agreed upon exclusively to only NPIL. Further, in this so-called knowledge partnership, one also gets to witness how financialisation of knowledge that is generated through public resources takes place and becomes *equity* in a commercial transaction.

Similarly, another PPP venture TCGA was established in the year 2003 by IGIB and a private-sector partner CMS. The stated objective behind the establishment of TCGA is to create the best infrastructure for use by R&D institutions, universities, and industry; act as a Technology Business Incubator (TBI); and develop human resources through hands-on training and provide accessibility to infrastructure on charge for service basis (CAG, 2013). This PPP project was put to a halt in 2011—eight years after its functioning—due to the unearthing of financial irregularities and mismanagement by the Comptroller and Auditor General (CAG) of India.[4] According to the report published by the CAG of India, the private partner in this collaboration has taken undue advantage of its public-sector partner in terms of infrastructure, resources, and finances. All of these irregularities were committed by the private partner through its non-profit subsidiary, Institute for Molecular Medicine (IMM). By virtue of IMM being a non-profit entity, it was provided incentives such as tax rebates by the Indian government. Taking undue advantage of this provision, the private partner has committed financial irregularities by merging the accounts of TCGA with IMM, ignoring the fact that TCGA in itself is a separate entity and is not a non-profit entity. In this process, the public-sector partner could never receive any share in the revenues that were generated by TCGA despite investing more than the private-sector partner in this collaboration. What is also interesting to note in this collaboration is that while the private-sector partner has committed to an investment of Rs 125 million, nearly three-fourths of this investment is committed towards building construction, the contract to which was awarded to another sister company of the private partner. On the other hand, the public-sector partner has invested Rs 135 million towards the project as an investment (CAG, 2013).

The undue advantage taken by the private partner can be further understood from the following instance. According to the CAG (ibid.) report, for the concept, design, and construction management, IMM involved its sister company, The Chatterjee Group Developments India Pvt Ltd (TCGD) through an agreement in the year 2004 for a total fee of Rs. 8.3 million. IMM agreed to pay 75% of the normal monthly fees—i.e. Rs. 0.15 million—in case the project was not completed in the stipulated timeframe of 18 months due to delay from their side. According to the CAG report (ibid., p. 69), there was a delay in the construction work of the building due to delays in receiving statutory approvals, but the agreed payment of Rs. 0.15 million was unilaterally increased to Rs. 0.3 million and Rs. 0.4 million, respectively, during December 2005 and February 2007. A total of Rs. 17.7 million was paid as a fee to TCGD, more than double the initially agreed upon Rs. 8.3 million by the end of 2010. In this context, the report notes that the private partner significantly diverted its capital investment through such agreements with its sister companies. There were multiple such acts by IMM during this whole project. As much as Rs. 5.3 million was written-off from TCGA during 2006 to 2007, 2009 to 2010, and 2010 to 2011 without the approval of any advisory committee (ibid.). The CAG report also noted that IGIB extended benefits to its private partner through providing land and expensive machinery, which the private partner used for purposes other than those involved with TCGA. The conflict of interest also sprung up because CMS had another subsidiary by the name of TCG Lifesciences (TCGLS) Private Limited, which was into performing global contract research and manufacturing. This firm was established in the year 2001, and one can safely assume that the high-end services offered by TCGA in order to support and build national capabilities were being deviated towards a favourite. In fact, in TCGLS's draft red herring prospectus that companies are mandated to publish before they go for IPO, it is stated that "we have an arrangement with the Institute of Molecular Medicine (founded by one of our Promoters), whereby we get access to The Centre for Genomics Applications, a facility for genomics and proteomics research located in New Delhi." (TCG Life Sciences Limited, 2007, p. 72). All of these details make IMM look more like a shell firm was established under the disguise of a non-profit entity to ensure that the profitable ventures of CMS are benefitted.

Both the cases of Genomed and TCGA clearly depict how private partners have taken undue advantage of public resources for their own benefit. While the rationale given for PPPs is that it does provide incentives to invest by risk sharing between the public and private partners, what one gets to witness in the aforementioned cases is the mere exploitation of public resources by private enterprises. In the case of Genomed, what one gets to witness is an exclusive monopoly over publicly funded knowledge to the private partner concomitant with diminishing autonomy of publicly funded institutions and financialisation of knowledge. Similarly, the case of TCGA is one of the testimonies of how such projects act in order to further the interests of private capital, while aspects such as innovation, national growth, and distributive justice remain rhetoric to masquerade the process of accumulation. Both of these cases also exemplify how Indian-origin enterprises take advantage of public resources as part of their accumulation process in a similar way that their global counterparts did negating the apprehensions of the neocolonial doomsayers.

The Private Way

This section provides a detailed description of the early days of the industrial endeavours of MBT businesses in the private sector in India. These firms carried out their business before there was an emergence of a stable ecosystem of MBT innovation in India. Although the GoI was offering several incentives for the growth of the MBT industry during this period, a stable ecosystem for biotechnology in India emerged only after NBDS-I, which is after the year 2007. Also, the firms that are being discussed are relatively successful in their business endeavours. Hence, an examination of the trajectory of these firms will provide an understanding of various factors that have contributed to their success. The firms discussed are Biocon, ARCI, Shantha Biotechnics, and SLiSc.

The reasons for discussing the aforementioned firms are as follows: these firms represent the beginning of the commercial MBT scenario in India in the private sector. Biocon is the first biotech company in India which shifted its business strategy from the initial idea of manufacturing enzymes using methods of molecular biology to a biopharmaceutical firm later. ARCI, established in Bengaluru, is a kind of TBI funded by the multinational Astra AB Pharmaceutical Limited. Shantha Biotechnics is the first successful biotech vaccine manufacturer from the country using rDNA technology. SLiSc is a classic case of a commercial establishment spin-off from the IISc and also the first scientific entrepreneur firm in India. Through the case studies of these firms, I attempt to decipher the role of several important political-economic actors and institutions that facilitated the rise of commercial MBT establishment in India before the emergence of an organised ecosystem.

Biocon: 'Managing' the State and Disregard for Organised Labour Movement

Biocon is the first commercial biotechnology firm in India established in the year 1977 as a 70:30 joint venture with the Irish-based Biocon Ltd (Singh, 2016). This joint project took place at a time when there was hostility towards foreign direct investments (FDIs) in the country with the then Janata Party not allowing more than 30% holdings by foreign entities (ibid.). Biocon has many firsts to its credit. It is the first commercially established biotech firm in India. It is the first firm in the biotech sector that went public. It is the first to get Food and Drug Administration (FDA) approval for a rDNA biosimilar. Biocon's journey was similar to some of the most successful DBFs in the US. It had investments in the form of VC and private equity (PE) and went for an IPO in 2004. This event marked the birth of a biotech billionaire in India. On 7 April, the day of its IPO, the shares got oversubscribed 33 times within five minutes of the opening. The share price crossed Rs. 500 and finally settled at Rs. 435, a 52% premium on the offer price of Rs. 315. The company was valued at 1.1 billion USD (ibid.). However, Biocon's success didn't lead to a quick spill over for the growth of the MBT industry. It took a lot of time after Biocon for any other biotech firm to go public. This is despite the fact that there have been a large number of incentives from the government for the growth of this sector.

Biocon started by manufacturing enzymes for its Irish firm, and after building resources and gaining capabilities, it went on to become a successful firm on its own in enzyme manufacturing. Understanding that the market for enzymes is limited, it ventured into the business of biopharmaceuticals (ibid.). Interestingly, the company's first product was insulin, but a biosimilar, the same one that Genentech—the first successful DBF in the US—manufactured as its first product. The company also established several subsidiaries over time in India and abroad to market their products outside India. In 1993, Syngene, a subsidiary of Biocon, was incorporated as the first CRO. The initial investment for this project came from a US-based firm which was looking to outsource its research (ibid.). Later, it established another subsidiary named Clingene, a clinical research wing that does clinical trials for large multinational pharmaceutical firms and also for its own pharmaceutical products. The idea behind establishing these different units covering various parts of the value chain of the drug manufacturing process was so that it would in turn help Biocon acquire capabilities to become a complete unit of drug manufacturing, as well as help in generating some revenues. The story of Clingene is very interesting to pursue. After global consulting agencies like McKinsey, Ernst & Young (EY), Frost and Sullivan projected huge growth in the clinical trial industry, a slew of CROs in India flourished during that period (IBEF, n.d.; Singh, 2016). But the projection did not manifest into reality and pushed most of them into losses (Singh, 2016).

One of the significant causes behind it was that, around the same time, a clinical trial disaster took place in India in a study of the human papillomavirus which killed seven tribal girls in a study sponsored by the so-called global non-profit agency PATH (Sunder Rajan, 2017). This led to a strong debate on the safety of the subjects recruited for the trials. The Supreme Court of India passed a judgement leading to a complete banning of the trials until the necessary mechanisms to ensure the safety of subjects were put in place. Also, the first amendment to the Drugs Act in 2013 that mandated compensation for injury and death during clinical trials was seen to affect the business as such. The industry was upset about the sweeping application of compensation for every death in a clinical trial without considering the cause of death (Singh, 2016). They claimed that between 2005 and 2011, around 3,000 deaths took place in clinical trials of which only 87 were attributed directly to the trial. However, health activists discarded this claim by saying that data of deaths were provided by the internal ethics committees of private companies and could not be relied upon (NDTV, 2017). As a result, in 2013, Clingene was merged with Syngene due to a drop in the clinical trial business followed by the IPO of Syngene in 2015 (Singh, 2016).

Most of the information I discuss here about Biocon comes from the book *Myth Breaker: Kiran Mazumdar-Shaw and the Story of Indian Biotech*. This book caught my eye at the Bioeconomy Conclave organised by the Association for Biotechnology Led Enterprises[5] (ABLE). The event was attended by several key people from academia and industry. To name a few present, there was the patent officer of the Indian Council for Medical Research (ICMR), a director of an IIT, CEOs of two of the biggest TBIs in Bengaluru, the business development head of IGIB, and several students from a local college. ICMR had a stall to market their research to the industry with video presentations and pamphlets. This book was presented as a gift to the speakers of the conference, who were mostly from academic institutes, marketing their research, and some start-up founders. Not surprisingly, the event took place at IISc in Bengaluru. To quote a few lines from the book, the marketing strategy of Biocon whose tagline is

> "Dynalix-Dynamic Helix" because "Biocon derives from Kiran's personality which is dynamic, bold and agile". The double stranded DNA structure became corporate logo, with a strap-The difference lies in Our DNA.
>
> (Ibid., p. 164)

Kiran Mazumadar-Shaw's dynamism and the difference in our DNAs sounds like a casual attribution of the so-called success to that of genetic determinism. The book is majorly a heroic construct of Kiran Mazumdar-Shaw, and while it does function that way, the riddles explained in that image construct also serve as a source to inform the corporate influence and how they resolve issues with the state. For instance, Biocon has a translational research centre at its cancer hospital. It was seeking Department of Scientific and Industrial Research's (DSIR) recognition for tax exemption. The department refused permission on the grounds that the R&D centre should be housed outside the hospital. However, according to the book, the centre got approval later because Ms. Shaw convinced the authorities that rule was misinterpreted. The directive was apparently only about the clear separation between a non-profit and commercial entity in operations and not in a physical location (ibid.). However, available research shows that the physical closeness between a non-profit entity and a for-profit entity "influence[s] an organization's access to sources of raw materials, employees or volunteers, and markets for its products or services" (Bielefeld & Murdoch, 2004). Today, Biocon's Mazumdar-Shaw Cancer Centre houses a translational research centre in the form of a non-profit entity that helps firms such as SLiSc where Kiran Mazumdar-Shaw has made a strategic investment (Singh, 2016).

Finally, the two successful products that Biocon was able to bring to market were in alliance with a Cuban biotech firm which she was initially hesitant to align with because of Cuba's communist polity. This kind of hesitance had its roots in the beginning days of Biocon when the firm was moving into a bigger facility at another place and as quoted in Singh (ibid., p. 29),

> Kiran wanted to promote local employment. Scores of people, mostly uneducated, were hired and they lost no time in forming a union. They shot off a letter to the management asking to be acknowledged as a labour union, without stating any problem that needed to be resolved. One morning, as employees walked in for work, it was shutters down; all local hires were sitting on dharna. They joined a communist labour union.... Nothing stopped, even for a day, but the lesson they learnt was not to hire *uneducated* employees. To this event Ms. Shaw retaliated by *automating* the plant.

While Biocon responded to the struggles of its employees and learnt not to hire any uneducated employees because of their affiliation with a communist movement, paradoxically, the irony being, it had to align with a Cuban biotech firm that possessed higher capabilities for technology transfer that could help bring its product to the market that Biocon boasts about even to this day.

ARCI and Globalisation of R&D

ARCI is a research centre and a kind of first TBI established by the multinational Astra AB Pharmaceutical Limited in Bengaluru as a section 25 company and non-profit society under the Karnataka State Registration of Societies Act. The ARCI case is very interesting for the fact that it is the first-of-its-kind institution for biotechnology in India. It was one of the two MNC R&D centres present in India even before complete liberalisation (Sharma, 2015). The reason behind ARCI's establishment in India is largely due to the infectious disease market here (Differding, 2017) and the availability of the necessary resources to perform R&D at reduced costs. Its initial collaboration was with IISc, which is a renowned public academic research institute and a leading molecular biologist of those times who was a professor at IISc played a crucial role in establishing this centre. When this professor was offered the opportunity to be the director of ARCI, he rejected the offer, saying,

> One has to realise that not all professors at the Institute are positively inclined towards research centres that have a connection with the industry. By staying back as a professor, I think, in the long run, I can influence other professors to see the positive side of this collaboration.
> (as cited in Singh, 2016, p. 75)

In fact, this professor was among the very few biotechnology scientists in the country at that time, and the availability of his research on a toxin for a mysterious neurological disease in North India to turn into a diagnostic was an initial point that convinced ARCI to start its project in India (ibid.). As Singh (2016) further notes, after the written permission for the establishment of the centre came from the government, deliberations took place between ARCI and the government about the constitution of the board, and it was decided that the board would have representatives in equal proportion from both the government and Astra Pharmaceutical Limited. However, there were a few issues that were to be sorted before the unit could become fully functional. In the meantime, the same professor (mentioned earlier) has helped ARCI to establish a unit in his laboratory at IISc, and six fresh PhDs were hired for this purpose. He was provided with a sizeable grant for building new laboratories by ARCI, which was subsequently rejected by the chairperson of the biological sciences division, and a local newspaper carried a front-page news report accusing the professor of planning to move the centre with some top-notch scientists to ARCI (ibid.). However, the centre was finally set up at a separate location but close to IISc on 7 January 1987 inaugurated by then PM Rajiv Gandhi. The centre has several distinguished scientists on its governing board, including a Nobel Prize winner. The governing board also comprised the stalwarts of Indian academia such as Prof. CNR Rao (IISc), Prof. Obaid Siddiqui (Tata Institute of Fundamental Research), Prof. G Padmanabhan (IISc), Prof. G. P Talwar, and Prof. K Banerjee (Ramachandran, 1991a). J. Rama Chandran, who was then a part of Genentech in the US, one of the most celebrated biotech firms at that time, was the first director of the centre. ARCI was established in India when Indian markets were yet to be completely liberalised. It looks like this is the reason why it was registered under section 25 as a non-profit entity. Being a section 25 company, though ARCI cannot itself make profits, it can involve itself in the projects of the multinational Astra AB in Sweden, and it did so in its early years (Reddy & Sigurdson, 1997).

It was a time when internationalisation and globalisation of R&D started taking place where MNCs started moving out of their home countries to developing countries, for one to develop innovations with the low cost of R&D infrastructure and capabilities that these nations possess as well as to capture local markets (Sharma, 2015; Reddy & Sigurdson, 1997). The establishment of ARCI in India should also be situated in the same context. According to its first director, J. Ramachandran (1991a, p. 533), "Astra's intent to organise a research centre in India was based on the scientific talent and competence available in molecular biology, bio chemistry and bio physics." Initially, ARCI started off with producing small enzymes and reagents that were being imported then. ARCI transferred this technology (a by-product of their ultimate aim of drug manufacturing for infectious diseases) to a company called Genei (Gene India) started jointly by a scientist from Tata Institute of Fundamental Research and a non-resident Indian scientist entrepreneur (Mytelka, 1999). ARCI has been a strong influence in the setting up of biotech start-ups in Bengaluru, one of the successful Indian cities in terms of biotech ecosystem. The prominent global strategy that was being followed in the biotech business then was M&A of successful biotech firms by big pharmaceutical firms. ARCI's assistance to start-ups in Bengaluru also cannot be delinked from its overall objective of marketing therapeutics in infectious diseases in India. Several successful start-ups today like Genei provide reagents and enzymes, including Xycton, which is into developing diagnostic kits; Gangagen, headed by Ramachandran himself, which is developing novel therapeutic proteins; and Bugworks (BW), which is into developing anti-microbial resistance drugs are all spin-offs from ARCI. In 1991, after liberalisation, Astra AB set up a wholly owned subsidiary named Astra Biochemical Ltd. to commercialise technologies developed by ARCI (Sharma, 2015). Eventually, after Astra AB's merger with Zeneca PLC as Astra Zeneca, ARCI became a part of it. Finally, in 2014, the centre was shut down when it saw that pursuing R&D in infectious diseases was no longer profitable (*BioSpectrum*, 2014; Differding, 2017).

The story of ARCI indicates that the multinational pharmaceutical firm was able to establish a TBI because of the strong support it received from IISc. The resistance towards the establishment of its laboratory in IISc also indicates the prevailing scenario of those times. However, Astra's intent to establish a research centre in India was because it wanted to enter into biotechnology, but rather cautiously through the use of resources available in India. While ARCI led to the growth of several biotech start-ups in India, the economic rationale behind such encouragement was the idea that successful innovation from these start-ups would provide an opportunity for ARCI to expand its business through M&As. On the other hand, with the government looking to encourage biotech business, and it being the very beginning of the Indian biotech industry, the possibility of building an ecosystem through ARCI may have led to the establishment of ARCI.

Shantha Biotechnics: The U-Turn Vaccine Nationalism

Shantha Biotechnics is a biopharmaceutical company that was into vaccine production. It is the first indigenous firm to produce the hepatitis B vaccine using the rDNA method. The firm was established in 1993 by Dr. Vara Prasad, who is a trained electrical engineer. As Dr. Prasad recounts, it was during his visit to a cousin who was a scientist in the Environmental Protection Agency in the US, whom he accompanied to a WHO conference on the impacts of immunisation in developing countries, that motivated him to establish this firm. In Prasad's words,

> [T]wo white people were making very derogatory comments, harsh comments, very unparliamentarily, not acceptable to normal civic people [such as], these beggars come with a begging bowl for subsidised vaccines, how long we should protect these beggars? They don't care about their children. Whenever there is an epidemic, they come with a begging bowl, they don't have their own program of immunisation, they don't develop their own vaccine and they say that they are poor. How long we have to carry this burden?
>
> (Prasad, 2019)

After returning from the US, Prasad set up the firm in Osmania University under the University Industry Interaction Programme (Shantha Biotechnics, n.d.). The initial capital required for establishing the firm came from his friends and family. Prasad was able to raise an amount of Rs 1.91 crore and registered Shantha Biotechnics (Prasad, 2019). Before this, Prasad met Dr. Anji Reddy, the founder of Dr. Reddy's Laboratories[6] about the starting of an rDNA project on hepatitis B. According to Prasad, Anji Reddy discouraged him saying that there was virtually no biotechnology in India, and it was not the time to venture into it (ibid.). This did not discourage Prasad, and he went ahead with the project. As Prasad (2019) recollects, the then vice-chancellor of Osmania University, Prof. Malla Reddy, encouraged him by providing him laboratory space free of cost in the university premises. An assistant professor from Osmania University helped Prasad in setting up this firm on the campus through her expertise and also by helping him recruit people. Prasad and the assistant professor struck a deal that Prasad would sponsor her travel to the US, and she would go there and learn technological know-how. She proposed the idea of working on interferon, a cancer drug, and Prasad added hepatitis B along with it. It was based on these two products that the university-industry alliance took place (Joshi, 2017). The professor went to the University of Missouri and started working with help from Prof. Guntaka Reddy in his lab. It was here that the idea to use *pichia-pastoris* as a host cell for rDNA came up instead of *e-coli* that was the prevalent system till then (ibid.).

A year after it began its stint in Osmania University, the firm had to move out because of "institutional politics" as put by Prasad (Prasad, 2019).

Later, it was moved to CCMB, where it was incubated for a year and a half. Shantha Biotechnics' presence in CCMB has helped it in a variety of ways. A scientific officer in CCMB who later joined Shantha says that CCMB provided "intellectual hand holding, scientific endorsement, infrastructural support and alignment" (Joshi, 2017, p. 126). In 1995, with the help of former PM Mr. PV Narshimarao, Prasad found an equity partner in the form of Oman's Foreign Minister H.E Yusuf Bin Alwai Abdullah, who infused 1.2 million USD for a 50% equity stake (Chakma, Masum, Perampaladas, Heys, & Singer, 2011). Abdullah had also facilitated a term loan of Rs. 15 crore from Oman International Bank at an interest rate of 4.75% when it was around 19% in India (Singh, 2016). In the same year, ICICI's United States Aid for International Development provided a loan of one million USD. With this money, in 1995, the firm moved to its own establishment with production facilities (Joshi, 2017). In 1996, the company received a grant of Rs 8 crore from the Technology Development Board (TDB) of the DST. Shantha, which started its operations in the year 1996, was the first company to receive this grant from the DST. In 1997, the company was able to bring a hepatitis B vaccine named Shavanac-B to the market at a price of one USD. At a selling price of one USD, the firm was able to make net profits of around 20% (Chakma, Masum, Perampaladas, Heys, & Singer, 2011). An important point to be noted here is that it was able to do so because of the process patents that were allowed then. At that time, the vaccine was patented by Merck for its plasma-derived hepatitis B vaccine and SmithKline Beecham for the rDNA vaccine. The two firms held a monopoly on the vaccine, and a single dose of the vaccine was as high as 23 USD. Dr. Prasad again approached Reddy Laboratories to market the vaccine for which Reddy Laboratories offered to market it for Rs 519, a rupee less than the MNCs. Shantha Biotechnics rejected this and went ahead with a new marketing strategy of mass immunisation campaigns with the help of the Indian Medical Association, All India Medical Council, All India Paediatric Association, district administrations, and local doctors (Joshi, 2017). These camps were held across India at a price of Rs 50 for adults and Rs 25 for children. This led to huge profits for Shantha Biotechnics. After Shantha's success, several domestic firms such as Bharat Biotech, Serum Institute, and Panacea Biotech ventured into the market, bringing down the price of the vaccine further lower to 0.23 USD (ibid.).

While Shantha had an expectation that its vaccine would be included in the UIP, and therefore a guaranteed buyback from the government, it took a decade more for the manifestation of this expectation. It is also important to note that there was a huge debate in the country then about the need for hepatitis B vaccine, given the ambiguity in the numbers about the prevalence of the disease in the country (Madhavi, 2013). While Shantha's innovation was turning successful, its MNC counterparts alleged that Shantha's product lacked quality and could therefore be toxic. This led to a quality comparison test ordered by the Drugs Controller General of India. The tests that followed had negated the allegations that were raised. Meanwhile, in 1999, the journal *Vaccine* published a study with findings that Shavanac-B was superior in its efficacy to others (Joshi, 2017). This study helped Shavanac find global markets and also helped in bagging UNICEF's order for supplying the vaccines (ibid.). In 2000, the company set up a subsidiary in the US named Shantha-West due to the inadequacy of clinical trial mechanisms in India (Chakma et al., 2011). In 2002, it received WHO prequalification status that helped get a brand image for its vaccines. In the same year, Shantha also received the help of Pfizer, the MNC pharmaceutical firm, to co-market its vaccine nationally and internationally (ibid.). Finally, in 2006, the company was acquired by a French pharmaceutical company, Mercuriex, which bought 60% of the shares but allowed the company to retain its name. In 2009, it sold its shares to Glaxo SmithKline at a valuation of 784 million USD, and now Prasad is a non-executive director of the company with 17% shares (Joshi, 2017).

In short, while BIBICOL's story is about how it became incorporated as a market for multinational products, the story of Shantha Biotechnics is a little different. Initially, it challenged MNC firms and took over their markets. This was largely possible due to the then existing patent regime of 'process patents' in India. Also, as we have seen in Prasad's words, the establishment of Shantha Biotechnics had an underlying nationalistic and salvationary rhetoric. In fact, when GoI introduced 100% FDI in the biotech sector, Prasad strongly criticised the government, saying that it was a "prescription for killing the local industry" (Jayaraman, 2005, p. 2). But ironically, Shantha Biotechnics ended up as a subsidiary firm of another MNC through an M&A, which is a very prominent corporate strategy of market expansion. The dissent that Shantha received during its early days in Osmania points to an unusual scenario of its time. It was only a matter of a decade[7] before such relations started to emerge in a more prominent manner, overcoming the initial dissent through policy aid from the state.

SLiSc: The First Academic Spin-Off and Its Complex Networks

The next case that is discussed here is SLiSc. SLiSc is also a unique company in India as it is a typical case of academic entrepreneurship and an exemplification of the rise of the scientific entrepreneur in India. SLiSc is also the first bioinformatics company in India. The company is a spin-off from IISc where four professors were the founders. It was established in 2000, the same year IISc had allowed its professors to engage in entrepreneurship activities by starting their own start-ups (Pulakkat, 2015). The initial impetus for the start of this company by its founders came when they were doing a sponsored research project for a US-based firm named Genomics Collaborative Inc (Biospectrum, 2003a). IISc had already established a section 25 non-profit company named the Society for Innovation and Development (SID) in 1991 to encourage entrepreneurship by providing mentorship, seed capital, and other resources (SID, n.d.). IISc had a policy of holding an equity share in the companies it incubates and SLiSc is a first instance of this (Ghosh, 2014). This process of sharing equity was started in the country by IISc even before the much commercially oriented CSIR did so (Pulakkat, 2015). It was also the time when Malsaekhar,[8] who was on a mission to re-orient CSIR into a commercial mode, introduced a new scheme for CSIR scientists to go out and set up a firm and come back in three years in case it did not work (Pulakkat, 2015).

SLiSc started by doing bioinformatics and developing platform technologies and later went on to do clinical genomics by sequencing and annotating individual genomes, thereby becoming a part of precision medicine. SLiSc growth took place in a typical way that happens with start-ups. It received its first round of funding from VC in the year 2001 from UTI ventures, an amount of 1.3 million USD (Ghosh, 2014) for equity of 17.5% (Business Line, 2001). A year later, WestBridge Capital Partners, a US-India VC firm, invested 1.9 million USD (Ghosh, 2014). A Japanese firm name MediBic also invested in SLiSc for a minority stake of 10%. It also received a fund of 0.9 million USD from ICICI's spread fund, 0.4 million dollars from CSIR's New Millennium Technology Leadership Initiative (NMTLI) and 1 million USD from TDB (Business Line, 2004). Altogether, SLiSc was able to generate 4.2 million USD in its first round of funding both from VC and angel investors. While the market for genomic tests in India was not so prevalent at that time, the investments seem to have come mostly due to the potential that the company has in serving the international markets (Biospectrum, 2003a) by developing platform technologies. This is evident from the fact that the company's first product idea that was pitched was for AVADIS,[9] a platform for data analytics in experimental biology applications (SLiSc, n.d.-b). The firm, before its second stage of funding, was also involved in doing contract research for many global firms, hinting at their business strategy of providing services for global customers (Bowonder & Mani, 2002). However, the company's first product that came onto the market was 'Soochika'—a software that helps analyse genomics data—in 2005.

This technology went on to become GeneSpring marketed by Agilent Technologies Inc (SLiSc, n.d.-a). Agilent is a US-based life sciences company that operates in the mode of business-to-business (b2b) transactions by providing services, instruments, and other facilities. SLiSc's initial business plan of doing bioinformatics and developing platform technologies for other biotech companies and pharmaceutical companies later got diversified. Its name change from Strand Genomics to Strand Lifesciences in 2005 points to this (genomeWeb, 2005). It diversified its business from just doing bioinformatics to developing platform technologies and ventured into several other operations. Currently, the company has operations in three different areas—namely, clinical diagnostics, bioinformatics, and clinical research. The company established a subsidiary in the US named Strand Scientific

Intelligence Inc for its operations there in 2010 (Business Wire, 2010). In 2013, in its series B of VC funding by Biomark Capital, a spin-off from Burril and Co, it received a funding of ten million USD. This deal involved buying the shares of previous investors, leaving Biomark Capital the only investor in its series B funding (Biospectrum, 2013). With the help of this investment, SLiSc launched its clinical diagnostic business. Strand's global market ambitions clearly become visible again through its act of establishing another subsidiary in the US named Strand Genomics in collaboration with El Camino Hospital in San Francisco for providing clinical diagnostic services (SLiSc, 2013). It started this service first for the US market and then in India. It also collaborated with a US-based innovator intermediary firm named Biohealth Innovation to expand its market there (Medical Laboratory Observer, 2014). In India, it was only in 2014 that SLiSc ventured into the clinical diagnostics business. It established connections with numerous hospitals across India, including Max Hospitals, Mazumdar-Shaw Cancer Centre, St. Johns Medical College Hospital, Kidwai Memorial Institute of Oncology, Health Care Global (HCG), and Apollo Hospitals (Ghosh, 2014) and currently claims to have such connections with over 300 hospitals in India (Quadria Capital, 2018). In fact, it has 20 genomics diagnostics labs spread across the length and breadth of the country (SLiSc, n.d.-a).

In 2016, the company tried going public (getting listed on the stock market), which eventually did not take place. Strand made a deal to acquire in a reverse merger fashion a penny stock company named Venaxis, which is listed in NASDAQ (Rai, 2016). A reverse merger, unlike a straight one, is when a small or low on performance company acquires a bigger company or one in profits. Generally, this takes place because companies can go public by skipping the first part of the process, which is the IPO. Singh (2016) observed that the pressure faced by Biocon by going public may have led to a change in decision by SLiSc. In 2018, the company merged with Triesta Sciences, a cancer diagnostics company which is a part of HCG, a leading oncology chain with a shareholding of 48.5% (Rai, 2018a). This merger seems to have been generated out of a business strategy to acquire the network of hospitals and market base that Triesta was serving. In 2018, after this merger, SLiSc acquired a strategic investment of 13 million USD from Quadria Capital, a PE[10] investor focused on healthcare sectors (ibid.). After this deal, the company also acquired the Indian subsidiary Quest Diagnostics Inc, a portfolio company of Quadria Capital (Dorbian, 2018).

The journey of SLiSc, which started from IISc till today where it is backed by PE has involved several actors including the state, academia, and VCs. It also indicates how complex these networks of production are. SLiSc was performing outsourced services in order to gain capital from foreign VC funds that could later help in the expansion of its markets. While it is a truism that speculative capital makes investments in riskier ventures, it need not necessarily mean that they do not indulge in risk reduction mechanisms. The journey of SLiSc to first venture into platform technologies was to prove to the VCs that it possessed the necessary capabilities to ensure returns on their investments. The support it got from IISc in the initial days and state funding from TDB and NMTLI also cannot be ignored. It is also important to note that SLiSc marked the emergence of a scientific entrepreneur spin-off from an academic space in India.

All the case studies discussed here are vignettes of only successful first-generation firms before an organised ecosystem for biotech was established in the country. Similar to the developments in the US, most of these firms had active support from state, academia, and finance capital. However, these relationships took place only at an individual firm level. This scenario started transforming in 2007 when the DBT introduced its NBDS-I, which paved the way for the establishment of an organised MBT ecosystem. The introduction of NBDS-I is a watershed moment in the trajectory of biotechnology in India. The following chapter focuses on how an organised ecosystem developed in India and what role the Indian state played in this process.

Notes

1 By neo-colonialism, Bhargava meant that India would end up depending on multinational firms.
2 Genomed has two units with one at the Institute for Genomics and Integrative Biology (IGIB) campus in New Delhi and the other associated with Well Quest, a Clinical Research Organisation (CRO) associated with Well Spring Hospital in Mumbai. All of these entities are seeded by NPIL. For details, see Sunder Rajan (2005).
3 Phramacogenomics is a technique used to rationalise the clinical trial process by classifying the trail subjects based on their genetic response to drugs.
4 CAG is a statutory body in India, which audits the GoI, the state governments, and the institutions that are fully or partially under central or state governments.
5 Kiran Mazumdar Shaw was a crucial force behind the establishment of ABLE and its first president. The establishment of ABLE preceded a long, drawn-out political battle between various groups in the biotech industry, eventually leading to separate lobbying groups for separate subsectors, with ABLE representing the MBT sector.
6 Reddy's Laboratories is a prominent and successful pharmaceutical firm in India.
7 Discussed in detail in Chapter 4.
8 Discussed in more detail Chapter 5.
9 AVADIS is a short form for Access, Visualise, Analyse, and Discover and is a platform designed for comprehensive data analysis and visualisation (SLiSc, n.d.-b).
10 The difference between PE and VC is that while PE investments go to mature companies, venture capital mostly goes into start-ups.

Chapter 2

MBT Ecosystem and Neoliberal State

The emergence of the MBT scenario in India, as discussed in the previous chapter, entailed a significant role of the state that was prioritising economic growth through private capital accumulation. However, this initial period lacked an organised ecosystem, mostly because, as characterised by the scientific elite and policymakers in the country, this was a period of learning. Alongside, during this period, the primary focus was on the information technology (IT) sector that was registering impressive growth rates for the country through its exports. With the crash of the global dot-com bubble during the early 2000s, there was a need felt for another sunrise sector similar to IT by the ruling class in India. This need for another sunrise sector can be captured through the words of former PM Mr Atal Bihari Vajpayee who stated that IT refers to India Today and BT—the acronym for biotechnology—refers to Bharat Tomorrow while unveiling a policy document in the year 2001 called "Biotechnology-A Vision-Ten Year Perspective." Before the implementation of this policy, the National Democratic Alliance headed by Mr. Vajpayee lost the election, and the United Progressive Alliance assumed the office. However, the focus towards biotechnology as an opportunity for economic growth and a new policy document charting the course of the development of biotechnology in the country for a period of ten years in the name of National Biotechnology Development Strategy-I were unveiled. The unveiling of this policy document is a watershed moment in the trajectory of biotechnology in India. The enactment of this policy enabled the state to become an active agent for private capital accumulation in the biotech sector in the country by providing various kinds of subsidies to the business class. It has extended support in terms of increasing budgets to the discipline of biotechnology in order to transfer the research results of publicly funded science to the private industry. Further, with this increased budgetary support to the DBT, new institutions, subsidised infrastructure, and capital support in terms of investments were all made available. While based on the theory of neoliberalism, the Indian state has put an end to subsidies that were being implemented in the interest of the poor and marginalised sections of the society, on the other hand, by enacting policies such as the NBDS-I, large-scale subsidies were being extended to the business class

DOI: 10.4324/9781003292104-3

to help them in their capital accumulation process. In fact, these subsidies in the form of NBDS-I were further intensified and extended by another five years through the NBDS-II unveiled in 2015. Additionally, the Indian state also has introduced policy reforms in several inter-related areas that are of direct interest to the business class in the biotech sector. This chapter critically discusses in detail all of these policy initiatives from the Indian state to subsidise the private biotechnology industry and thereby demonstrates the neoliberal character of the Indian state.

Increased Budgetary Support

Biotechnology in India has received preferential treatment from the state. The Ministry of Science and Technology, which is the nodal agency to promote science and technology (S&T) in India, before DBT, had only two other units—i.e. DST and Department of Scientific and Industrial Research (DSIR)—under it. The special preferential treatment provided can be witnessed from the fact that before the establishment of DBT, the budgetary allocations to S&T were divided between DST and DSIR, which are like the umbrella organisations of S&T in India. But after the establishment of DBT, the budgetary allocations were divided between DST, DSIR, and DBT, and biotechnology was the only sub-discipline that received this kind of treatment. In the initial year of DBT's establishment, DBT's share of the total S&T budget was 12.4%, which peaked close to 25% between the years 2010 and 2015 (see Figure 2.1). The average share of DBT of the total S&T budget between 1986 and 2019 is nearly 20%. In Figure 2.1, if we look at the trend lines with respect to budgetary allocations, we can witness that the trend line of DST is more or less constant, while DSIR is declining and that of DBT is increasing.

It is also important to point out here that neither DST nor DSIR is restricted from using budgetary allocations for biotechnology-related projects. Even by any conservative estimate, if at least 5% of budgetary allocations of DST and DSIR are going towards biotechnology-related projects, on average, it received at least 25% of the total budgetary allocation, vindicating the preferential treatment by the state. Such generous sanction by the state is because it believes that the "macroeconomic issues of the country are associated with this science's development." In the US as well, where the biotech phenomenon first originated, the successful private commercial biotechnology establishment preceded a substantial increase in budgetary allocations to the discipline of life sciences (discussed in the introduction; AAAS, 2018). It is for a similar reason that biological sciences in India also received such preferential treatment.

Figure 2.2 indicates how budgetary allocations started increasing steeply during the period 2002–07 and further increased by more than three times in the corresponding next five-year period. These periods of high budgets are also associated with significant milestones in the trajectory of DBT,

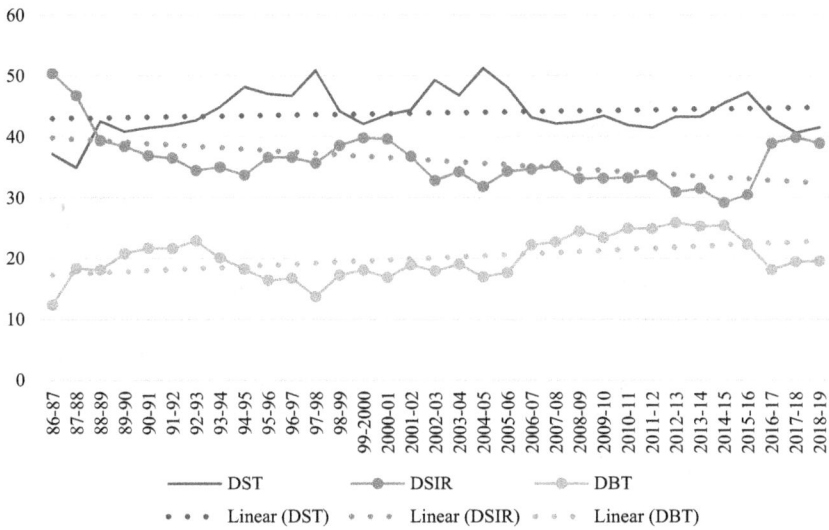

Figure 2.1 Percentage Share of DST, DSIR, DBT in Total Budget Share Allocated to S&T

Source: Author's compilation from budget documents, GoI (https://indiabudget.gov.in/previous_union_budget.php).

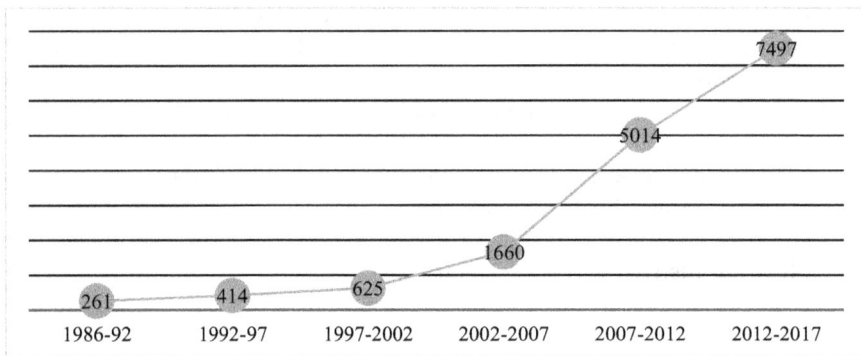

Figure 2.2 Budgetary Allocations to DBT during Five-Year Plan Periods.

Source: Author's compilation from budget documents, GoI.

especially the period during 2007–12, where there was a sharp increase in the budgetary allocation to DBT.[1] As a part of this strategy, DBT committed 30% of its budgetary allocations to PPPs (DBT, 2005).

Institutional Support

With increased budgetary support over the years, DBT has established several new autonomous institutions. DBT currently has 15 such institutions, and more than one-third of DBT's budgetary allocations go to these institutions. Another large chunk of budgetary support goes towards extramural projects for universities, national research laboratories, scientific and industrial research organisations, and the corporate sector. For 2014–15, the latest year for which data with regard to expenditure on extramural projects is available, DBT spent nearly 40% of its total budgetary allocation on extramural projects (DST, 2018). In the same year, DBT's autonomous institutions have accounted for more than 35% of DBT's total expenditure (DBT, 2016). These figures indicate how these two categories dominate the overall DBT expenditure. However, what is important to note here is that these allocations are associated with the objective of encouraging market-led biotechnology endeavours. Although India tried to have a policy in the form of the Protection and Utilisation of Publicly Funded Intellectual Property Bill, 2008, similar to the Bayh-Dole Act in the US that led to the commodification of knowledge by allowing publicly funded research to be commercialised, the Bill was withdrawn due to strong opposition from civil society. However, the objective with which the Bill was introduced was achieved in the following way. For instance, DBT, which spends a huge sum of money towards its autonomous research and extramural projects, allows the sponsored institutions to hold complete rights of the patent and licensing deals and keep the revenues to themselves. This is exactly the same function that the Bayh-Dole Act did for US universities. It allowed universities to commercialise their research results that were federally funded. By letting these institutions keep revenues to themselves, DBT incentivises them to vigorously patent their innovations. This is explicitly stated by the DBT in the following instructions issued for technology transfer and IPR:

> With a view to encourage the institutions to file patent applications on their innovations, motivate them to transfer their technologies for commercialisation, and facilitate them to reward their inventions, the following instructions are issued.
>
> (DBT, n.d.-d)

DBT believes that "intellectual property… has become a crucial driver of economic growth" (ibid.). However, since patents are not just scientific or technological in nature but techno-legal entities in a commercial transaction, new institutions such as TTOs have come into existence in order to guide these institutions and market the research. In fact, DBT in its NBDS-II resolved to create 150 TTOs across the country with an objective "to strengthen industry-academia collaboration and facilitating process of transfer of research leads and technologies developed at research organisations and academic institutions to relevant industries for further product development and commercialisation" (DBT, 2018, p. 4).

Another important institution to discuss is BIRAC, established in 2012 by the DBT to take care of all the PPPs and industry-related biotechnology matters in India. The pace of biotechnology in India picked up, particularly during the period of the 11th five-year plan period. During this period, the budgetary allocation to DBT increased by more than three times as compared to the previous five-year period (see Figure 2.2). It was also the period when DBT initiated PPPs in order to propel the bioeconomy by committing 30% of its budgetary allocation towards this cause in its NBDS-I (Jayaraman, 2005). As a part of this commitment, DBT initiated two PPP programmes—namely, the Small Business Innovation Research Initiative and Biotechnology Industry Partnership Programme—by providing capital to biotech firms in the form of soft loans and grants. With increasing budgetary allocations, the industrial focus of DBT was further augmented, and in 2012, DBT established a non-profit section 25 company named BIRAC to help propel biotechnology entrepreneurship. A senior level officer from BIRAC explains the functions of BIRAC as follows:

> Identify innovation, handhold innovation and how to protect that innovation and take that innovation so that it becomes commercially dearest to the funders and by protecting the IP and things so that it becomes like a planned development. Not only funding, we thought we should bring—in funding parlance—360-degree management of innovation where funding plays a role and also take care of the scientific challenges. When science is not good, how much ever funding you have, your innovation does not work. Similarly, business plan development, your exit strategy and regulatory issues all play a critical role. So we thought we should push each of these elements apart from funding. Take innovation to a level where it becomes commercially dearest, it can walk, it can be licensed out. BIRAC created six months back a unit called product commercialisation unit. It works across funding cycles for any project which is now funded by BIRAC but needs a push for hand-holding to the next level not only in terms of funding but IP, technology management, connections, policy implications etc. This project is very close to the heart of our secretary. Her instruction to us is to identify innovations which require not only funding but other help as well and take it to the next level. BIRAC will also help in finding potential licenses.
>
> (Source: Personal Interview with BIRAC representative)

The road map for BIRAC for the decade following its establishment was prepared by ABLE (DBT, 2012). ABLE is the lobby organisation of biotech firms established in India in 2003 that negotiates with the state for the necessary favours. Even today, most of the statistics with regard to the industry put forward by DBT are based on the findings of ABLE (BIRAC[a], 2019). In India, industry lobbyist organisations participating in policy making started with liberalisation when then PM Rajiv Gandhi took the support of the Confederation of Indian Industries (CII) in 1986 for the opening up of the economy (Athreye & Chaturvedi, 2007). Scoones (2003) points out how in the case of Karnataka, scientific elites and corporate leaders dictated the biotech policy of the state. Similarly, ABLE was able to induce the state in order to have a favourable policy environment. If we look at the recommendations provided by ABLE to BIRAC in 2012, we understand that the trajectory of BIRAC has been in the same direction over the time period. There are five core recommendations relating to easing the regulatory policy, increasing university-industry interlinkage, TTOs, TBIs, promoting entrepreneurship, and providing risk capital and tax incentives. While how these recommendations are put to practice is seen in the previous sections, in the following sections, we examine how BIRAC's trajectory has been set by ABLE. Das's (2015) critique of the new economic policy (NEP) in India provides insights into the processes through which industry organisations set the official agenda of research and development. He states,

> NEP is the neo-liberal program of the bourgeois class first, and a government policy second. To the extent that neo-liberalism is a government policy, it represents a "wish-list" of the big business which gets a sympathetic hearing from the pro-market state managers.
>
> (Ibid., p. 716)

This is further vindicated by the fact that ABLE only represents big biotech businesses while it claims to be a representative of the whole of the biotech sector in India. It is important to highlight here that not even a single respondent of the five biotech firms interviewed as part of the fieldwork conducted at a TBI in Hyderabad said anything substantial about ABLE, and some of them did not even know what ABLE is. For instance, a senior science policy researcher who is also a member of several committees constituted by DBT, when asked about ABLE, responded as follows:

> It's an industry body, but I am not sure that it lobbies for startups. I think it lobbies for slightly older companies and all. It definitely keeps the biotech industry visible to the centre but I don't know, you should ask startups, but none of them have ever talked to me about what ABLE has done for them. None of them, not once. So that makes me a little suspicious that it may be not serving the purpose of the startups.

A start-up in Hyderabad, also relatively successful, when enquired whether they know about ABLE, responded as follows:

> Yes. They always invite us for some programmes, but never interacted or took any policy suggestions from us.

Another start-up founder responded to a similar question as follows:

> No, [I don't know]. Is ABLE something which connects technologies with VCs or other companies?

All this evidence makes one question why DBT and BIRAC are dependent on ABLE in order to guide them for policy and also to implement the same. In fact, recently in November 2019, DBT hosted the Global Bio-India summit on a large scale as a part of which it released the Indian-Bio Economy Report 2019, which is largely based on statistics and policy directions provided by ABLE. In one sense, these evidences make it difficult to differentiate between state institutions DBT and BIRAC from the lobbyist organisation ABLE.

Infrastructure Support

In order to ensure that the innovations of biotechnology guarantee market returns, there is a need for critical infrastructure. Again, this is a trend witnessed from the so-called successful nations' biotechnology paradigm. Particularly in the context of biotech, it was witnessed that innovations take place in a cluster environment. A cluster environment consists of all the actors required for carrying on the innovation concomitant with the market activity. A typical biotech cluster in the US consists of universities, public research institutes, and legal actors to protect intellectual property (IP), supporting firms and industries along with financial resources. Imitating the same model, the government also invested in developing similar clusters in India. According to DBT,

> Research and development in the biotechnology sector in a cluster format with core emphasis on innovation is critical for the growth of biotechnology entrepreneurship. Keeping in view the importance of developing bio-clusters, National Biotechnology Development Strategy aims to establish India as a world-class bio-manufacturing hub by creating a technology development and translation network across the country through the establishment of bio-clusters, incubators, technology transfer centres etc.
>
> (DBT, 2020)

There are currently six operational[2] biotech clusters in India, and the GoI plans to establish four more.[3] While most of these clusters are established by the central government, a few of them have been established by the state governments as well. For example, the biotech cluster in Hyderabad was established as a part of the initiative of the state government of Andhra Pradesh (AP) to encourage biotech entrepreneurship. According to a CEO of a leading biotech cluster, elements of a biotech cluster include R&D institutions, TBIs, biotech and pharma companies, fiscal incentives and VC investments, and other infrastructure (see Figure 2.3).

The elements mentioned earlier also indicate a biotech firm's external relations of production essential for its effective functioning. But what is even more important to notice is that almost all of these resources are put in place through public money and the active involvement of the state. This is in sharp contrast to the laissez-faire principles propagated by the neoliberal theory wherein the state is supposed to stay out of market activities for its

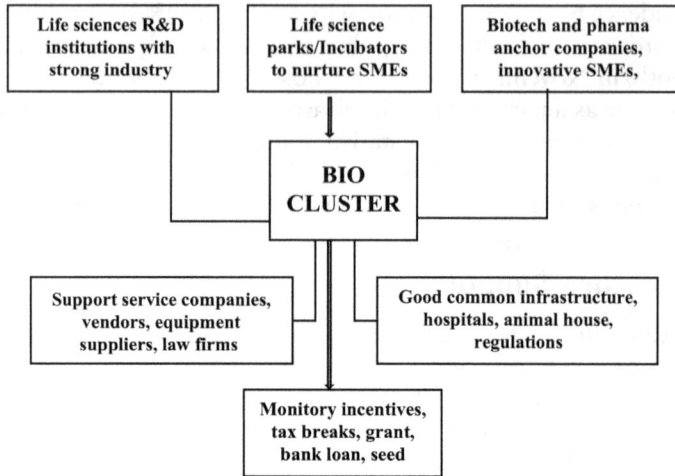

Figure 2.3 Elements of Biocluster.

Source: Based on Chattopadyay, n.d.

efficient functioning. Instead, what we witness here is the active involvement of the state in order to provide resources for private activity far below the market price of these resources. One of the important components of these clusters is the presence of TBIs. In India, currently, there are nearly 50 TBIs supported by DBT's BIRAC with a commitment of Rs 213 crore (BIRAC, 2020a). Most of these bioincubators are generally associated with host institutes which are primarily public academic centres that can give access to their laboratories, equipment and expertise. The rationale provided by BIRAC for providing public resources at subsidised costs to private ventures is that biotech innovations are highly risky in nature and make VCs reluctant to invest in early stage projects. And also since biotech ventures need a space with high-end R&D facilities, BIRAC through its schemes fulfils these needs (ibid.). The other forms of infrastructural support include biotech parks established by the DBT in association with other government organisations. Currently, DBT is a part of nine such parks in various parts of the country. In 2019, DBT came up with the National Biotech Park Scheme to accommodate the graduated start-ups from incubators, again with subsidised resources. This scheme calls for PPPs and state governments, along with a private partner, to establish biotech parks where DBT would provide 75% of the project cost and the state government provides the land (DBT, 2019b). Sunder Rajan (2006, p. 89) characterises the ideology behind the establishment of Genome Valley in Hyderabad—a PPP between the state government of AP and ICICI, which is a financial service company—in a similar kind of process where the park provides a subsidised environment to the start-ups as "intervention of no intervention" premised on the neoliberal ideology of minimal state intervention, "an ideology that, in order to be upheld, requires massive state intervention." Additionally, the GoI also offered various subsidies to big corporate houses in the name of Special Economic Zones (SEZ). According to the Ministry of Commerce, there are currently five biotech SEZs of which four are held by private companies and one in PPP (Ministry of Commerce, 2019). The private-sector SEZs are Serum Bio-pharma park, Biocon, Shantha Biotechnics, and Frontier Life Line, and under PPP is Genome Valley in Hyderabad. However, Serum and Biocon are the top bio-pharmaceutical firms in India with a revenue of nearly Rs. 5,000 and Rs. 4,000 crore in a year, respectively (*BioSpectrum*, 2019). Shantha Biotechnics has been acquired by the multinational pharmaceutical firm Sanofi Aventis.

Capital Support

Capital is one of the most critical elements that is required if at all the envisioned idea of entrepreneurship is to be manifested. In several countries such as the US and Israel, as well as European countries, which had a successful stint in fostering the entrepreneurship phenomenon, the state played a definite role by providing some kind of risk capital in the form of grants to early stage start-ups (Owen, North, & Bhaird, 2019). Another and most important source of capital for these start-ups is VC, which is supposed to be completely a private industry affair. In the Indian case as well, state support to the MBT sector in the form of grants is enormous. In fact, VC activity in the biotech sector did not pick up the momentum like in countries such as the US, and the state took the responsibility to fill this gap. Several agencies of the state such as DST; Ministry of Micro, Small, and Medium Enterprises; and CSIR provide the risk capital required to the start-ups. However, for biotech start-ups, DBT and BIRAC have become major sources of support in terms of capital requirements. BIRAC till 2019 has supported over 650 start-ups (nearly one-fifth of total biotech start-ups) with a funding of Rs 1,162 crore (BIRAC[c], 2019). It provides capital support in terms of grants, equity, and soft loans in order to support the biotech firms at the various stages they pass through. To quote the version of BIRAC,

> BIRAC's funding mechanism encompasses the entire range of the product development pipeline—from ideation to proof of concept to later stages including validation, scale-up and commercialisation.
>
> (BIRAC, 2015)

The capital support to the industry is also extended by the state participation in the VC market either by investing in several private VCFs or by establishing its own VCFs, which is further discussed in detail in Chapter 3.

Favourable Policy Environment

The favourable treatment from the state to the biotechnology sector is a result of the macroeconomic policy decision subsequent to economic liberalisation in India. As mentioned in the previous chapter, biotechnology was seen as an opportunity for economic growth in the liberalised free-market economy which India committed to in 1991. While one can definitely argue that such favourable treatment has also been received by the IT sector in India, one should also not forget that it was for the same reason that the IT sector was prioritised (Upadhyaya, 2004). Both the IT and the biopharmaceutical sectors are viewed as the largest export-oriented sectors. NBDS-I states, "[B]iotechnology can deliver the next wave of technological change that can be as radical and even more pervasive than that brought about by IT" (DBT, 2005, p. 3). Although the initiatives from the state to encourage the biotech sector began in the late 1980s and early 1990s, the whole of the decade between 1990 and 2000, there was not much significant commercial activity. Several leading scientists from the discipline categorised the decade as a learning experience (Padmanabhan, 2003). In order to ensure that the sector contributes to economic growth, several steps have been taken by the state. In 1995, according to a news item that appeared in *Science*, new rules were introduced to push scientists towards the industry (Anonymous, 1995b). These rules were introduced because most of the products brought into the market from public laboratories failed. According to the report, the new rules necessitated that the work conducted should be world-class, involve collaborations with the industry, and be patentable. While the news report provides no evidence with respect to the implementation of the new rules, it does provide the emerging ideology of biotech policymaking.

Thereafter in 2001, DBT unveiled a vision document with a ten-year perspective. This new vision document focused on various issues. It called for the funding of research projects which are time-bound and utility-based, encouraging PPPs to bring products to market, and easing of regulatory measures through a single-window clearance policy for biotech products (Anonymous, 2001). Encouragement of IPRs was also a part of this vision document. In the same year, GoI announced 150% tax rebates on R&D spending by private industries (Jayaraman, 2001). After this vision document, several states in India developed their own biotech policies in order to encourage the industry through various fiscal and regulatory incentives (Chaturvedi, 2002). Several biotech parks started coming up due to these initiatives by the state. The reason that states in India took biotech so seriously was because they believed that biotechnology could help them ride another economic wave similar to IT. For example, in AP, the then chief minister Chandrababu Naidu introduced Andhra Pradesh-Biotechnology policy in 2001, which provided several incentives to the industry. It reduced the sales tax on high-end biotech products, which ranged between 8% and 16% previously, to just 1%; built biotech parks for providing subsidised space to the industry; and proposed to have an exclusive biotech fund of Rs 500 million (ibid.). The State of Karnataka, which previously had a Department of IT, converted it into the Department of Information Technology-Biotechnology. Similar developments took place in most other states as well. However, the first-ever national policy on biotechnology in India was NBDS-I drafted in 2005. While there was a vision document already for a ten-year period, the biotech industry pressurised the GoI to introduce a national biotechnology policy similar to the National Information Technology Policy. In 2003, the biotechnology industry association pressurised then DBT secretary for a national policy. The DBT secretary, disagreeing with the proposal, responded that "there is no requirement for separate biotechnology policy" (BioSpectrum, 2003b, p. 3).

However, due to strong pressure from the industry, the new national policy draft was put out for consultation in 2005 and implemented in 2007 (Newell, 2007). With the first national policy in place, DBT has set the trajectory of the industry by providing the necessary means. One of the central objectives of NBDS-I is, "with the introduction of the product patent regime, it is imperative to achieve higher levels of innovation in order to be globally competitive. The challenge now is to join the global biotech league" (DBT, 2005, p. 5). It is through this policy document that all the industrial needs such as human resources, infrastructure, tax and fiscal incentives, academia-industry interaction, FDI policy, and PPPs have all been institutionalised. This policy document calls for 30% spending of all public funding along with private partners (Jayaraman, 2005). It also provided several fiscal and trade incentives, such as exemption of import duty, removal of customs duty on imported material, and tax deduction on R&D to even patent filing expenditure (DBT, 2005). The establishment of a large number of biotechnology parks and incubators as a priority with incentives for firms established in those centres is a result of this policy measure. Financial support to private firms in the form of grants and soft loans was all initiated as a result of this policy. Under this policy, 100% FDI is allowed by the government in the sector (Jayaraman, 2005). This raised serious apprehensions among the domestic industry leaders. For example, Dr. Vara Prasad of Shantha Biotechnics who brought out a low-cost hepatitis B vaccine expressed the view that 100% FDI is a "prescription for killing the local industry" (ibid., p. 2). Ironically, a few years later, Shantha Biotechnics was acquired by a big multinational pharmaceutical firm. After the announcement of NBDS-I, the biotech ecosystem grew significantly in India.

In fact, it is no exaggeration to say that before this policy, there was no such thing as a 'biotech ecosystem.' After this policy document, in 2015, DBT brought out NBDS-II with further enthusiasm. While in NBDS-I, universities were seen as potential sites for human resource development, NBDS-II called for redesigning of universities for evolving an ecosystem to "nurture" scientists, innovators, and entrepreneurs. The NBDS-II had more or less similar guidelines like NBDS-I, of course in a much more intense manner, but it differs in one crucial aspect. NBDS-II talks about entrepreneurship in a big way. The word 'entrepreneurship,' which appears just once in the draft NBDS-I, appears 25 times in NBDS-II. In fact, the title of NBDS-II is itself '[p]romoting bioscience research, education and entrepreneurship' (DBT, 2015). This idolisation of entrepreneurship, however, was initiated before this policy document. The establishment of BIRAC as a non-profit organisation by DBT is specifically for the promotion of entrepreneurship. While in the NBDS-I, only one financial assistance programme for small and medium enterprises in the name of the Small Business Innovation Research Initiative was proposed, currently, there are more than ten financial assistance programmes run by BIRAC to support biotech enterprises (www.birac.ac.in). Unsurprisingly, this enhanced focus on entrepreneurship is just the tip of the iceberg of the large-scale neoliberal turn that was taking place in the realm of India's political economy. While policy measures to implement neoliberal austerity and private capital accumulation were in function pertinently after economic reforms, the rise of knowledge economies demanded further intensification and implementation of the core neoliberal principles. As a result, the GoI, in order to unleash the "individual entrepreneurial freedom" (Harvey, 2005, p. 2), initiated a programme called Startup India in 2016. The objective of this initiative was to ensure that start-ups sprung up in large numbers. In order to implement this objective, several measures and incentives were put in place by the state. Large-scale tax concessions, self-certification with regard to the implementation of labour and environmental laws, fiscal and trade incentives, financial aid, and subsidised infrastructure were all put in place (GoI, 2016a). BIRAC was made an implementing agency for this programme in the biotech sector.

The developments in the biotech sector followed a more or less similar strategy like in the case of IT. In the case of IT as well, large-scale deregulation, fiscal and tax incentives, human resource development combined with infrastructure support resulted in the growth of the industry (Arora & Bagde, 2007). However, while the IT industry also needed skilled manpower, it did not lead to the establishment of large-scale research institutions. This is because the IT industry was performing mostly backend services. But biotech demands very highly skilled manpower and advancements in R&D given that biotech ventures are very risky, particularly drug development. Additionally, while the Indian biotech industry also engages in large-scale backend operations at the lower end of the value chain, this is not a very viable option for the industry as such. This is because the Indian consumer markets were previously entirely dominated by domestic capital before the globalisation and harmonisation of patent laws. In order to secure these markets, it is important for the industry to have access to high-end R&D capabilities. This is the reason why the two policy documents by DBT emphasise the need to enhance human resources by initiating biotechnology programmes across all the universities and research centres in the country and by also announcing special fellowships for students pursuing research in the area of biotechnology. The setting up of autonomous research institutes is also largely due to this need. India becoming a signatory of WTO and ratification of the TRIPS Agreement is another major policy breakthrough that necessitated a strong R&D infrastructure in order to become competent in the global pharmaceutical and MBT industry and market.

While the product patent regime was implemented in India against the wishes of industrial organisations such as the Federation of Indian Chamber of Commerce and Industry (Muzaka, 2018), India did not enact a national policy on IPR till recently. It only had patent rules implemented by the Department of Industrial Policy and Promotion and a Patent Act that was amended from time to time. Due to severe resistance from civil society organisations and last-minute bargains by the left parties during the United Progressive Alliance (UPA-I) regime, several relaxations[4] were provided by the state in the implementation of the Patent Act (Sunder Rajan, 2017). There was constant pressure from MNCs on the Indian state for the removal of these relaxations enacted for public health measures. Even the US government put serious pressure on India with the threat of sanctions (Joseph, 2015). Yielding to this pressure, in 2016, GoI unveiled its first national IPR policy to create awareness about IPRs as a "marketable financial asset and economic tool" (GoI, 2016a). Marketable financial asset implies that IP can be traded like any other tangible property in the real estate market in a similar speculative fashion. The policy document also talks about IP as a collateral asset to raise loans from the banks. This is a principle already in practice in industrialised countries (Deshpande & Nagendra, 2017). Basheer and Agarwal (2017, p. 6) in their critique of the policy call it a one-sided perspective on IP "aimed at capturing its 'financial value.'" The most regressive measures in the policy document appear in the steps to be taken towards the objective of the generation of IPRs (GoI, 2016a, p. 8). Two steps particularly with regard to the publicly funded research are as follows:

• Encourage researchers in public-funded academic and R&D institutions in IPR creation by linking it with research funding and career progression.
• Include IP creation as a key performance metric for public-funded R&D entities, as well as technology institutions, and gradually extend such evaluation from Tier-1 to Tier-2 institutions.

The policy document in one sense coerces[5] the scientists in public-funded institutions to patent their research.

Notes

1 The year when DBT announced its first NBDS-I strategy
2 Bangalore, Hyderabad, Pune, National Capital Region, Chennai, Kolkata and Gujarat, Faridabad.
3 Faridabad, Haryana, Bangalore.
4 Pre-grant opposition, post-grant opposition, and Section 3 of Indian Patent Act, 1970.
5 This is further discussed in the chapter.

Chapter 3

Venture Capital

In the previous chapter, the role of the state in MBT ecosystem has been discussed. In this chapter, another important constituent—i.e. the role of finance capital, particularly in the form of VC—is discussed. If we look at the rise of the MBT industry in the US, it coincided with the large-scale deregulation of financial markets in the early 1980s (Roth, 2000). Muzaka (2018) argues that this coincidence is not mere happenstance but rather closely interrelated. Similarly, several other scholars have critically examined the role of fincanicalisation in MBT innovations in the global context. For instance, Mirowski (2012) argues that under the financialised model of innovation, MBT start-ups resemble something like a Ponzi scheme where firms typically do not produce any products or services. Developing it further and in contrast to Mirowski, Birch (2017) argues that under the financialised model of innovation, MBT firms resemble a reverse Ponzi scheme where the late-stage investor accrues the highest returns or nothing and vice versa. Further, Birch (2020) argues that under financialisation, innovation itself is problematic where its social promise takes a backseat. While there is much scholarly attention towards financiaisation of MBT innovations in the global context, the Indian scenario does not picture in these accounts. In fact, it is not yet clear whether there is a finacialisation of MBT innovations in India. The only critical enquiry that examined this aspect in the Indian context is Kaushik Sunder Rajan's (2006), celebrated work *Biocapital* where he characterises VC—the predominant form of finance capital under which biotech innovations take place—as speculative capital. From a Marxist standpoint, he differentiates between commodity capital and commercial/speculative capital. Commodity capital is that capital where capital circulation takes place through the production of commodities which are then sold in markets for the realisation of surplus value. Speculative capital on the other hand is capital for which circulation is an end in itself and need not be involved in the direct production of commodities. The speculative capital is put aside from the surplus that is generated through the circulation of the commodity capital. Sunder Rajan explains,

> Commercial capital, according to Marx, does not create surplus value
> in and of itself but does so indirectly by constantly perpetuating the

DOI: 10.4324/9781003292104-4

circulation of capital and by providing it with its own self-perpetuating, self-sustaining logic that does not need to originate from the moment of production of commodity.

(Sunder Rajan, 2005, p. 21)

For Sunder Rajan, speculative capital becomes a distinctive marker in analysing the frameworks of capitalism in India and the US. According to him, in the US, there is a dominance of circulation of speculative capital in the biotech industry, while India is yet to witness VC activity.

Depending on the institutional and legal structure within which these companies operate, one or the other of these forms can predominate in the creation of value; yet neither of these forms flow seamlessly from the other. And therefore in India, for instance, there has tended to be a more direct correlation between therapeutic molecule production, sales, profit margins and the value of a pharmaceutical company. In the United States, where biotech companies are almost always enabled by venture capital funding, and where biotech and pharmaceutical companies almost always become publicly traded companies when the opportunity presents itself (and therefore answerable to investors on the Wall Street), valuation is more directly dependent on speculative capital.

(Ibid., p. 21)

While Sunder Rajan argues that in the Indian context there is yet to witness the dominance of speculative capital, writing in a different place, he clarifies that, given the limited circulation of VC in India, the state took upon itself the responsibility to provide this capital to emulate the US start-up culture. According to the theory of Biocapital, the Indian state in itself became an active VC investor unlike its counterpart in the US where it is largely left to private investors. Based on this distinction, the theory distinguishes between the nature of the state in India and the US and thereby the relationship between capitalism and MBT.

"The state, therefore, has itself decided to provide VC, by setting up a fund to which the contributors are the Andhra Pradesh Industrial Development Corporation Ltd., the Small Industries Development Bank of India, and the AP Industrial and Infrastructure Corporation Ltd (see Naidu, 2000, p. 139). In other words, Naidu set up a system of public investment as "venture capital" funds, a completely oxymoronic conception of VC, which by its American definition comes out of huge private investment funds that expect an extremely high return on investment. Naidu's "venture capitalism" is, effectively, a euphemism for government subsidy for high-tech industry".

(Sunder Rajan, 2006, p. 8)

However, the current scenario of the relationship between MBT and VC in India puts to question the findings put forward by the theory of Biocapital. Also, a much deeper analysis suggests that the role of the Indian state in setting up VCFs is not entirely different from its global counterparts, including that of the US. In fact, it appears that it is based on the experience of the US that Indian policymakers made a case for state intervention to set up publicly funded VCFs. These are the two aspects that this chapter engages with. Whether there is an active circulation of VC in India or not, who are the agents of this circulation and is it is entirely different from the US scenario? In the following section, I look at the evolution of MBT and VC industries in India and juxtapose these two to understand the extent of VC circulation in the MBT industry and what this scenario is going to look like in the near future. Thereafter, I argue that the state intervention in India through the setting up of VCFs is not significantly different from its global counterparts. I also in turn argue that while the Indian state has actively engaged in setting up VCFs by itself initially, of late, it encouraged a different approach in the form of PPPs rather than it setting up its own VCFs. This is not to say that this approach is entirely new but evolved into a dominant form only in the recent past, hinting at the emergent relationship between VC and MBT in India.

VC and MBT in India

In India, the framework for the regulation of VC emerged only in 1996. Therefore, the story of VC in India needs to be examined starting from this deregulation exercise of 1996, which the theory of Biocapital doesn't fully take into account. After this deregulation exercise, there were significantly increasing investments of VC over time across the sectors. This deregulation is largely a result of the success of Non-resident Indians (NRI) entrepreneurs from Silicon Valley in the US and their interest in investing in IT ventures in India (Upadhyaya, 2004; Gonzalo & Kantis, 2017). However, as Scoones (2003) points out in his work on the development of the biotech sector in India, the Indian ruling classes believed that biotechnology is the next sunrise sector similar to IT. This is due to the crash of the global IT dot-com bubble in the early 2000s. Around the same time, there was also a kind of hype that was being generated and the rise of some local stalwarts of the industry as the torch-bearers. For example, Kiran Mazumdar-Shaw, one of the biotech stalwarts, was dubbed by *The Economist* as "India's biotech queen" (Newell, 2007). A senior science policy researcher and a close associate of BIRAC described the hype created around biotech and how biotech became a buzzword in India as follows:

Kiran has pushed the word biotech a lot. She has created this industry conceptually; like "we are the biotech industry".... There was a creation of this discourse around biotech which then gives her prominence and her company prominence. Then they set up an association ABLE and they set up Bangalore Bio which now is morphed into tech summit, and then she is called the biotech queen.

(Source: Personal interview)

Though the biotech phenomenon in India began in the late 1980s and early 1990s, only a limited number of DBFs ventured into MBT business activity, and it was the established pharmaceutical firms that were diversifying their businesses (Arora, 2005; Konde, 2009). It was only in the last decade, particularly after the setting up of an ecosystem with the active involvement of the state, that the biotech sector started booming in India with an increasing number of independent DBFs, as well as start-ups. This is unlike the growth of the IT industry in India which by and large was independent of the traditional business communities (Upadhyaya, 2004). The Indian biotech ecosystem today comprises start-ups, small and medium enterprises, and big firms. By the end of 2018, there were 2,669 biotech start-ups in India, of which 969 (35%) were established in 2018 itself, with a majority of them in the biopharmaceutical sub-sector (BIRAC[a], 2019). According to the estimates by the GoI, this start-up number is expected to grow further by more than four times by 2024 (ibid.). There are also 600 core biotech companies that are currently functional in India (ibid.) of which more than 300 are in the biopharmaceutical sub-sector (*BioSpectrum*, 2019). The Indian biotech sector is currently valued at 52 billion USD, and it aims to reach 100 billion USD by 2025 (BIRAC[a], 2019). The biotech business in India comprises four sub-sectors. They are biopharmaceutical, bioagri, bio-IT and services, and bioindustry. Biopharmaceutical is the leading sub-sector with about 54% of the revenues. There is also a strong bio-IT and services industry in India which contributes nearly 14% of the revenues (ibid.). In terms of sector-wise start-ups, it is again the biopharmaceutical sector that dominates, with over two-thirds of start-ups in the biopharma and diagnostic sector (ABLE, 2020). Of the 54% revenues generated by the biopharmaceutical sector, 50% is contributed by diagnostics and medical devices, 30% by vaccines, and the rest by biotherapeutics (BIRAC[a], 2019). Given these developments in the biotech sector in India, as well as a flourishing VC industry that has evolved from the time of its deregulation, it becomes imperative to revisit the claims of the theory of Biocapital in terms of the dominance of speculative capital. From the experience of countries like the US (explained in the introduction chapter), the role of financial actors in the innovation network of MBT is well established. For the MBT start-ups, VC has become an important source of funding in order to execute their ideas with innovation potential.

Before we further proceed towards examining the status of VC in the MBT ecosystem in India, it is important to understand the different stages that a start-up passes through and the general mode of functioning of VC. A start-up generally starts with an innovative idea. At this stage—generally referred to as the ideation stage—the investment required is called seed capital. This is the riskiest stage in the start-up cycle, and during the beginning of the MBT phenomenon, in the US, VC investors were investing at this stage (Hughes, 2011). However, in India, mostly, this seed capital is provided through various sources, such as friends and family, government grants, or the savings of the founders. Specifically with respect to MBT, GoI has stepped in, and through DBT's BIRAC in the name of the Biotechnology Ignition Grant (BIG), started providing such funding. At least one-fifth of the start-ups in the biotech sector currently in India received their seed funds through BIG (BIRAC[a], 2019). Using these funds, once the start-ups come up with a prototype, they approach VCs for investments, which is considered the growth phase. The VCs, along with investing for equity, also provide mentorship to the firms, and in some instances, they are a part of the management board.

VCF is a fund generally set up by high-net-worth individuals or investors or financial institutions or corporate firms. VC is also referred to as risk capital. This is because the ventures in which this capital is supposed to be invested in are risky in nature, either ensuring a high rate of returns in the case of success or a loss in the case of failure. It is also believed that VC is necessary because traditional financial institutions such as banks do not generally fund high-risk ventures. Particularly in the MBT sector, given the complex nature of biological mechanisms, the risk is even higher, and by that logic, the higher the necessity of VC. Hogarth (2017) explains that, generally, VCs expect a return on investment of 500%–1,000% over a period of five years. However, they also know that one-third of the investments will not yield any return, and one-third will only yield modest returns (ibid.). Navigating through these complex dynamics is how speculative capital functions in real time.

The logic underlying this relationship between the start-ups and VCs is that in case a start-up has a successful exit, the rewards would be mutually beneficial. But the VCs know that depending on a single venture for returns is highly risky, and hence they invest in a portfolio of companies. Even while investing in these portfolios, they ensure that the risk they are taking on is minimised. This is the reason why VC funding comes in rounds. Each round of funding is dependent on the 'milestones' that a firm achieves, which in turn increases the valuation of start-ups. There may be multiple VCs or a single VC which might participate in a given round of funding. While VCs in their early days did invest in riskier projects—i.e. even at the seed stage or the ideation stage—with time, they have evolved certain mechanisms to reduce the risk that they take on. One mechanism that has evolved over time in general, and more importantly in MBT, where products generally take a longer period, is the valuation of firms. These valuation techniques determine the value of a firm, taking into account several parameters, of which the most important is the future rate of earnings, generally referred to as discounted cash flows in accounting terminology (Birch, 2017).

In India, though there was VC activity during the early 1980s, it operated with very little scope, with mostly public institutions taking part (Bowonder & Mani, 2002). This initial VC activity was carried out by the state through public financial institutions. Thereafter, through the intervention of the World Bank (WB), the private VC industry also came into prominence (Dossani, 1999). However, after economic liberalisation in 1991 and with the rising prominence of the Indian IT industry, the need for VC was realised. In 1993, an organisation called Indian Venture Capital Association (IVCA) was established as a result of the initiative of NRI entrepreneurs to represent the interests of the VC industry (ibid.). Carol Upadhyaya (2004) explains in her work how multinational capital flows took place in India in the form of VC from Silicon Valley in the US. She mainly points to the role of NRIs, particularly those that made fortunes in Silicon Valley behind the upsurge of the VC industry in India. With the emergence of IVCA and as a result of their lobbying efforts, the Indian state in 1996 initiated deregulation of its financial markets (Gonzalo & Kantis, 2017) and made the Securities and Exchange Board of India (SEBI) a single nodal agency to regulate these funds, removing the earlier barriers in the form of multiple regulatory oversights from the Central Board of Direct Taxes and the Reserve Bank of India (RBI), along with SEBI. However, the 1996 deregulation exercise allowed foreign VC investments only for NRIs or through domestic VC units. In 1998, 80% of VC investment in the country came from foreign sources (SIDBI, 2019). After the 1996 regulations, on the recommendations of the K. Chandrasekhar[1] committee, in the year 2000, the regulatory framework of VC was further liberalised. The recommendations of this committee removed the restrictions previously applicable on foreign venture capital investors (FVCIs) and were allowed to directly invest in ventures of their choice (SEBI, 2003). This deregulation exercise also entailed several incentives to VC investors, with the most important being a "tax pass", where the VCFs are only taxed at the investor level and not the fund in itself, which was previously not the case (ibid.; SEBI, 1999). Thereafter, a series of amendments were made from time to time to further liberalise the financial markets. In 2006, the Technology Innovation and Venture Capital committee recommended further deregulation of the VC industry. It called for allowing pension funds to be invested in VCFs and also recommended that VC lending be recognised as priority sector lending by the GoI (GoI, 2006). Further in 2012, in order to further simplify the private investment scenario in the country, SEBI introduced the Alternative Investment Fund Regulations, 2012. In 2016, the Pension Fund Regulatory Development Authority of India allowed pension funds to be invested in VCFs (Dhanjal & Sarkar, 2016).

After several such deregulation measures, the current status in India, as per the SEBI data, is that there are 189 India-based VCFs and 254 FVCFs (SEBI, n.d.-a; SEBI, n.d.-b). Most of the foreign VCs route their investments through Mauritius to avoid double taxation. As per the data available with SEBI, till 31 March 2017, Rs. 74,889 crores of VC investment have been made in India, of which 75% of the funds came from foreign sources (SEBI, n.d.-b). Between 2008 and 2018, VC investments in terms of the number of deals in the country increased at a composite annual growth rate (CAGR) of 13%, while the amount of investment during the same period increased at a CAGR of 15% (SIDBI, 2019). In fact, between 2013 and 2018, the value of investments increased at a CAGR of 30%, which is more than double the overall period between 2008 and 2018 (ibid.). Of late, there are also increasing investments from domestic sources (ibid.).

If we look at the evolution of the VC industry in India, according to a report by the Small Industry Development Bank of India (SIDBI), it took place in three different phases. The period between 2000 and 2010 is characterised as a nascent phase, followed by the scale-up phase between 2011 and 2014, and thereafter the evolution phase. During the nascent phase, the report states that the investors were "testing the Indian waters" and set up funds to take advantage of the emerging start-up scenario in the country. The scale-up phase is defined by the aggressive VC competition due to the growing number of start-ups in the country, and the evolution phase is defined as VCs being selective about the attractive opportunities, with a focus on the quality of deals rather than the number of deals. Figure 3.1 shows the overall trends in terms of the number and value of deals between 2008 and 2018. Particularly, in the context of the biotech sector, according to data by SEBI, cumulative investments till 2017 are Rs. 425 crores, of which nearly two-thirds are contributed by the FVCIs, which is just 0.65% of total VC disbursements in the country (SEBI, n.d.-c). If we also add the share of the pharmaceutical industry to this, it becomes 1.4%. However, biotech, pharma, and healthcare together had a total investment of 7.7% (ibid.).

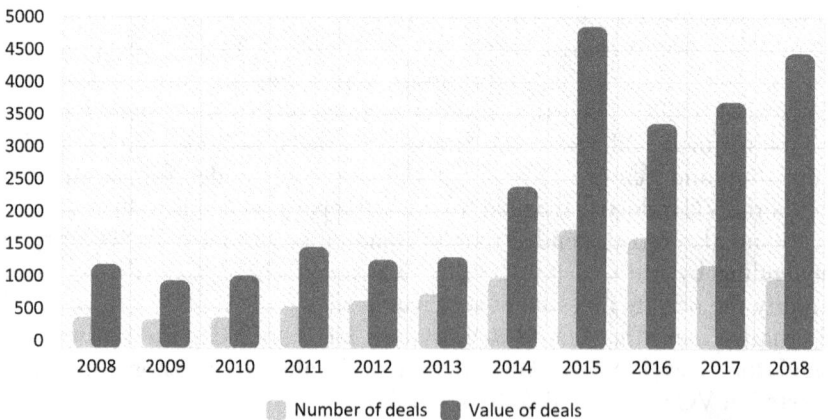

Figure 3.1 VC-Number and Value of Deals (Millions USD) between 2008 and 2018.
Source: SIDBI, 2018.

Now, given these facts, and by juxtaposing the developments in India's MBT sector, as well as the VC industry, the important question that needs to be addressed is, can the distinction made by Sunder Rajan (2006) in terms of the dominance of speculative capital still hold good in analysing the frameworks of capitalism? The answer is both yes and no. From the information available, one cannot deny that there is an active VC investment scenario in India. While it is true that VC investment in the MBT sector occupies a very small share; nevertheless, total investments show an upward in growth year on year (SIDBI, 2019), and there is a great possibility that these trends may also reflect in the MBT sector. This is because of the ongoing exponential growth in the number of start-ups in the MBT sector in the country through the active involvement of the state. This increasing number of start-ups will further lead to an increase in the number of start-ups entering the growth phase and thereby providing more avenues with lesser risk for the active circulation of finance capital.

The Indian State and VC

In this section, the discussion focuses on the role of the Indian state in VC disbursement and whether it is significantly different from its global counterparts. As mentioned already in the previous section, the Indian state has actively set up its own VCFs when it realised that there is a lack of VC investment scenario in the country. But if one closely looks at the roots behind such initiatives, it appears that there is no significant difference in this practice from elsewhere across the globe. For example, Dr. Y V Reddy (1998), a former governor of RBI, in his speech "Venture Capital and Technology Development in India," deploying the case of the Small Business Investment Company Programme of the US, which is a government-sponsored programme initiated for investing in technology-based companies for exchange of equity argued for similar initiatives from the Indian state.

In India, the first company to start a VC scheme was the Unit Trust of India, which is a statutory public-sector investment institution (DST, n.d.). Thereafter, India has witnessed several state governments establishing VCFs by themselves in order to fund start-ups. The State of Gujarat and erstwhile AP in the early 1990s started VCFs with assistance from the WB (Reddy, 1998). In 2003, the AP government initiated a first-of-its-kind VCF entirely focused on biotechnology (Financial Express, 2013). However, of late, the Indian state started taking a different approach in terms of its investments in VCFs. While during the initial phase, public institutions have actively set up VCFs, of late, what one gets to witness is a kind of PPP model of investments where public institutions are investing in private VCFs based on the risk-sharing principle. This form of risk-sharing arrangement, although it existed right from the beginning,[2] became a predominant form only recently. The recent initiative of India's flagship start-up programme launched in the year 2016, where a Rs 10,000 crores fund of funds managed by SIDBI was set up to invest in SEBI-registered private VC funds (SIDBI, 2019). Particularly with respect to the biotech sector, BIRAC was made a nodal agency to invest these fund of funds in private VCFs in the name of the Accelerating Entrepreneurship (AcE) fund. The BIRAC AcE fund is structured in such a way that it uses this fund only in combination with other SEBI-registered private VC funds (BIRAC, n.d.). The AcE fund is invested in what are called AcE daughter funds set up by private VCs with a clause that they contribute twice the amount contributed by BIRAC. These initiatives hint that they are designed less with the intention of profit-making by the state and more to ensure the presence of a missing element in the ecosystem which ultimately only benefits both the private biotech firms and VCs by reducing the risk that has to be taken on. Even in the case of the US, similar policies[3] were designed to stimulate private-sector investments (Cromwell Schmisseur LLC, 2013). This is not just the case of the US but also most European countries and countries including Canada, Australia, Israel, to list a major few, have the state establishing its own VCFs or investing in private VCFs (Owen, North, & Bhaird, 2019). This then makes it clear that the VC investments by the Indian state are not significantly different from the country's global counterparts, as stipulated by the theory of Biocapital. The capital support should not be seen as an isolated measure from the state but rather in relation to other measures it is taking in order to propel the private MBT industry.

Notes

1 A successful NRI entrepreneur from Silicon Valley.
2 For example, Technology Development Board, which is a public institution established in the year 1996 under the aegis of the DST, invests in several private VCFs that fund technology start-ups in the form of a PPP (DST, n.d.).
3 State Small Business Credit Initiative enacted in 2010 to provide federal funding for state-managed VC programmes which can in turn enhance private investment.

Chapter 4

Indian Academia.inc

Science and Technology (S&T) are accorded with a significant prominence in the development trajectory of the modern world, and India is no exception to this. The Indian state, right from Independence, accorded substantial importance to S&T (Visvanathan, 1998). It has established several publicly funded research laboratories (PFRLs) and universities to pursue scientific R&D in order to address social and economic needs. One of the objectives behind such generous sanctions was to ensure that the country becomes self-reliant through industrial progress. To meet this need, it was deemed necessary that S&T play a significant role. During the Independence movement, and immediately after it, there were two schools of thought as to what kind of development model the country should be adopting. On the one side was the Gandhian idea of improving the small and cottage industries and thereby reducing poverty and unemployment (Chibber, 2003; Frankel, 2005). On the other side was the developmental model put forth by Nehru of heavy industrialisation aided by the growth in S&T. After Independence, the Nehruvian model was put in practice, and to this end, S&T was accorded the highest prominence.

After Independence, for around four decades, at least ideologically, there was a division of labour with regard to scientific endeavours that universities should be concerned with basic research and PFRLs with applied research (Krishna, 2001). However, both of these institutions were not limited and confined to just those activities, and there was always an overlapping of the type of research that was performed by these institutions. The importance of scientific R&D for industrial development is well acknowledged across the globe and so too in India. But, given that the institution of science and its practitioners are supposed to be largely autonomous (Merton, 1973), there was always a question of to what extent the business world and the world of science should interact. This question becomes even more pertinent in the case of scientific institutions that are publicly funded and profit-making industries. The scholarly debates with such concerns can be broadly classified into three different categories. First is those who argue that though scientific R&D, especially in the academic spaces, has historically been away from the market, now its integration into market structures is nothing but inevitable

DOI: 10.4324/9781003292104-5

(Etzkowitz, 2003). The second group, on the other end of the spectrum, are those who argue that scientific institutions should be autonomous and engage in science for its own sake, and what is being currently witnessed is a collapse of scientific ethos and the rise of post-academic science (Ziman, 1996; Sunder Rajan, 2012; Slaughter & Rhoades, 2004). The commonality between these two strands is the assumption that scientific R&D was never influenced by external agents and is a phenomenon of the contemporary. The third category of scholars argue against such monolithic history that such an ideal science never existed and point to the periods of external agencies influencing the research agendas (Bernal, 1965; Kleinman & Vallas, 2001).

Keeping aside briefly the question about the historical influences on scientific R&D, it is important to note that scientific knowledge in the contemporary economic landscape—often termed as the knowledge economy—has become an important means of accumulation in various modalities (Birch, 2017) and articulations (Sunder Rajan, 2006) with several new characteristics. Given, currently, the complex forms of the articulation of knowledge at the same time as a means of production, a commodity, and a rent-deriving asset, there is a resurfacing of the question about the desirable extent of the relationship between publicly funded science and profit-making industry. Coming back to the question of the influence of research agendas by external agencies, it cannot be denied that historically, there were always periods of influence of external agencies in determining the research agendas. For example, during WW-II, the research agenda in most American universities was influenced by military funding, and even before that, there was the active participation of large philanthropic organisations like the Rockefeller Foundation and several other big conglomerates which were funding R&D in the universities (National Science Foundation, 1982). After WW-II, there was a steep decline in funding from these agencies and the state became the chief patron of scientific research in the US universities (ibid.). During this period, universities and scientists were structurally autonomous, allowing them to carry out their own research activities.

The contemporary scenario, conversely, is a radical departure in the sense that today there is a corporatisation of academic institutions with corporate cultures and mechanisms spewing across all the academic spaces. The dominant ideology that arose after WW-II that universities should maintain a distance from the market in order to retain their autonomy and engage in critical thought is becoming fast disoriented, with universities becoming increasingly integrated into the market structures. This ideology of staying away from the market is being replaced with a corporate ideology dominated by corporate managerial practices. Knowledge, which was once common and free-flowing is restricted and circulated in carefully curated channels. There is also an increased bureaucratisation of the university and the emergence of new audit cultures that were previously only associated with corporate entities (Sunder Rajan & Leonelli, 2013). The arising of such a phenomenon vis-à-vis *corporate managerial practices dominating the university, carefully curated channels of knowledge circulation, and different modalities of articulation of knowledge* is variously articulated as the arising of the entrepreneurial university, (Etzkowitz, 2003), venture science (Sunder Rajan, 2012), academic capitalism (Slaughter & Rhoades, 2004), etc. Much of this phenomenon, which started in the US, later traversed across the globe. There is also a coincidence of the occurring of this phenomenon with the rise of the molecular biology-based paradigm in life sciences (Pisano, 2006; Blumenthal, Gluck, Louis & Wise, 1986).

An entrepreneurial university is typically characterised by the following attributes.

a. Industry sponsoring research
b. Scientists acting as consultants to the industry
c. Technology transfer
d. Scientific entrepreneurs
e. TBIs

While there is ample literature that looks at the entrepreneurial university and examines its characteristics and consequences in the global context (Shapin, 2008; Hackett, 2014; Sunder Rajan, 2012, Slaughter & Rhoades, 2004; Slaughter & Leslie, 2001; Etzkowitz, 2003; Viale & Etzkowitz, 2010; Etzkowitz, 2013; Kleinman & Vallas, 2001; Vallas & Kleinman, 2008; Radder, 2010), any literature that demonstrates the corporatisation of Indian academia is lacking. This chapter attempts to fill this gap by demonstrating the processes of corporatisation of Indian academia and its characteristics. It is important to highlight here that a large number of universities in India are publicly funded, although there is an emergence of privately funded universities of late, particularly after the introduction of structural adjustment programmes in 1991 (Tilak, 2014).

This chapter begins by providing a detailed description of the characteristics of the entrepreneurial university in India concomitantly with the evidence of its corporatisation and the process of normalisation that follows. It also examines whether this corporatisation is a phenomenon that arose with the advent of biotechnology like in the case of the US (Pisano, 2006; Blumenthal, Gluck, Louis, & Wise, 1986). In order to demonstrate this, it is important to understand historically how the relationship between publicly funded scientific R&D and private industry has evolved in the country. This becomes important because, in India, there are a variety of institutions that are publicly funded other than universities that engage in scientific research, and most importantly, these institutions are quasi-academic in nature. They are PFRLs, Indian institutes of technology (IITs), IISc, Indian Institute of Science Education and Research (IISER), etc. PFRLs are established by various scientific agencies such as CSIR, DST, DBT, etc. In the following sections, a detailed description of the evolution of the relationship between publicly funded R&D and private industry is provided in order to explain the corporatisation of the university for the following reasons:

a. In the Indian context, though there is an ideological distinction between the functions of universities, PFRLs, IITs, etc. (university-like institutions), in reality, all of these institutions are involved in similar kinds of functions. All of these institutions pursue both basic and applied research, train students, and award degrees.
b. The corporatisation phenomenon initially began with the PFRLs and later got normalised in an incremental manner.
c. It was the so-called success of PFRLs, particularly the CSIR, in terms of corporatisation, that later encompassed all the academic spaces.

Given these reasons, it becomes imperative to explicate the interaction between PFRLs and private industry in India historically. Also given the short history of independent India, one can say that there is no disjuncture with respect to academia-industry interaction for R&D. However, one can definitely witness a shift in the nature of this interaction over time. In this chapter, I show that in the time period between 1947 and 1991, which is the period after Independence and before rigorous market liberalisation, the nature of interaction is of a different kind as compared to the nature of interaction that followed after liberalisation. The interaction during the pre-liberalisation period is more of a demand-driven one, while the one after liberalisation is neoliberal in character. The neoliberal time period can further be characterised in two ways as the Conquest of Innovation period between 1991 and 2015 and the Coercive Innovation period from 2015 which is still ongoing. The neoliberal characterisation is because of the following reasons:

1. implementation of *supply-side* measures and integration of academic spaces into the market structure,
2. rise of *entrepreneurial culture* in general and particularly in academic spaces and among academic scientists, and
3. corporatisation of academic spaces with corporate culture spewing across the academic spaces and the concomitant replacement of previously *non-market-oriented academic value system* with the *corporate value system*.

In a demand-driven environment, the type of interaction between academia and industry was one that is dominated by demand from the private industry. During this period [1947–91], the dominant modes of interaction were scientific consultancy and sponsored research projects. In a supply-side interaction, what takes place is knowledge production, *anticipating the arising of demand*—i.e. the interaction here depends not just on current demand but also on the *probability of the arising of future demand and thereby piling stocks of knowledge in the form of aggressive patenting*. The universities and academic spaces form a part of the supply chain by ensuring that there is a seamless supply of inputs for industrial production. This kind of interaction in India can be mapped during the period of economic liberalisation, which also coincides with the rise of the knowledge economy, prominence of innovation, and the biotech phenomenon. It is during this period that corporate culture crept into universities with separate marketing entities such as TTOs, universities participating in business activities for equity stake, rewarding employees based on the economic potential of their research, replacing the previously predominant non-market academic value system are all introduced. The third type of interaction, which is the period of Innovation 2.0, is the period of normalisation of this corporatisation. In order to normalise the corporatisation of academia, new mechanisms are introduced by the state to ensure that the wave of corporatisation sweeps across all the universities and even small colleges that are never provided with enough resources. It is during this period that rigorous assessment is done based on the extent of corporatisation that took place in the university/institute and naming and shaming of those that fail to get incorporated.

The following section discusses the historical nature of the interaction between public funded science and private industry in India with a special focus on the corporatisation of academia with respect to biological sciences. The chapter particularly focuses on PFRLs established by the CSIR and DBT, as well as IISc, IITs, and universities. This is because CSIR laboratories were the first to implement commercial measures in the country, and it was their success that prompted other institutions to follow. The corporatisation in DBT institutes is examined because of their focus on biotechnology. IISc and IITs are considered to be the best-in-class academic institutes in the country where commercial exchanges were in place right from their origin. All of these commercial measures later got incorporated into the university structure.

Demand-Driven Interaction—Independence to Economic Reforms Period

In India, right from Independence till today, the state has been the chief patron of scientific research. Till the beginning of the last decade, almost 75% of total R&D expenditure came from the state's exchequer (see Table 4.1). While after Independence there has been an increase in R&D spending as a percentage of the gross domestic product (GDP) over the years, of late it has stagnated at around 0.8% (Principal Scientific Advisor, 2019). This scenario is quite different from the other countries such as the US, China, and East Asian countries like South Korea which spend around 2% of their GDP on R&D (ibid.). The government, right after Independence, focused on establishing a successful relationship between the PFRLs and the private industry. This focus has only increased with time, with several macro changes in the global economy, thereby encompassing all institutions of higher education.

In India, higher educational institutions are divided into four categories. They are central universities, state universities, deemed universities, and institutions of national importance. Although the difference between these

Table 4.1 Percentage of R&D Expenditure by Public and Private Sources

S. NO	Year	Government Expenditure on R&D (%)	Private Industry Expenditure on R&D (%)
1.	1970–71	89.55	10.44
2.	1975–76	88.12	11.87
3.	1980–81	84.13	15.86
4.	1985–86	87.82	12.17
5.	1990–91	86.16	13.93
6.	1995–96	78.25	21.74
7.	2001–02	76.47	19.32
8.	2005–06	67.5	28.30
9.	2010–11	62.38	32.1
10.	2015–16*	56.09*	40.03*
11.	2016–17*	54.24*	41.95*

Source: DST (2018).
* indicates estimates by DST
Note: Expenditure for higher educational institutions is excluded.

different types of higher education institutions is not clearly defined, the Ministry of Human Resource and Development (MHRD) categorises all of them in two ways as university and university-like institutions. In the years immediately after Independence, the important state-funded research organisations that engaged with private industry were only the CSIR laboratories, IITs, and IISc (Bhattacharya & Arora, 2007). The most common types of interaction during this period were sponsored research and consultancy, which are demand driven in nature; endowment and philanthropic funding; and technology licencing to a limited extent. In the following subsections, a detailed overview of the type of interactions these organisations carried out is provided with respect to each of these institutions during this demand-driven interaction period.

CSIR

CSIR, which was previously known as the Board for Scientific and Industrial Research (BSIR) was established in the year 1940. The need to become self-sufficient in British India due to import cuts during WW-II in 1939 led to its establishment (Singh, 1986). In 1942, BSIR was transformed into CSIR. After Independence, the new Indian government continued with CSIR for the general progress of S&T in the country and also to perform R&D that could be put to use by the industry (ibid.). In its first five-year plan, recognising the importance of S&T for economic development, a chain of 11 PFRLs was established under CSIR to carry out industrially useful R&D, which increased to 40 with time. The first plan document, pointing out the role of S&T, states that, "for scientific research to make its full contribution, it is necessary that the results of laboratory work should be utilised in actual practice by being translated into commercial products" (Planning Commission, 1951). While the first plan emphasised the establishment of new institutions for promoting industrial research, the second plan emphasised strengthening the existing institutions and co-ordinating research in all national laboratories in order to upgrade the industrial and technological progress of the country. To meet this need, the National Research Development Corporation (NRDC) was established in 1953 to bridge the gap between R&D and to ensure maximum practical utilisation by industries (Planning Commission, 1956). The second-plan document also recognised the importance of universities as the main source of supply of competent and trained "scientific workers" (ibid.). Much of the state's focus on industrially oriented R&D is also because of the industrial policy adapted by it. Till 1991, the Indian economy was a closed economy, and the policy of import substitution only allowed import of those materials and technology that could not be availed in the country. However, the scope of imports varied across the time between 1947 and1964 and 1964 and 1991(Aggarwal, 2001). Initially after Independence (1947–64), given the model of development was towards the building of heavy industries, the import policy was more liberal in allowing technology transfers and FDIs. This liberal import policy later got tightened due to the foreign exchange crisis, bringing forward the goal of self-reliance with more vigour (Sandhya, Jain, & Mathur, 1990; Aggarwal, 2001). To this need, it was expected that CSIR would play a significant role.

However, with time, it was witnessed that CSIR could not contribute as expected towards the growth of industrial research in India. Right from its first review committee, CSIR was heavily criticised for not being able to perform as expected. The basis for this criticism was that in the years immediately after Independence, virtually all industrial R&D was carried out by CSIR (Desai, 1980). Thereafter, there was a significant drop in the industrial R&D carried out by CSIR because of the reluctance of the large industries to put to use technologies developed by CSIR (Valluri, 1993). This resulted in CSIR serving only small and medium enterprises. The decreasing trend of industrial activity led the third review committee of CSIR in the year 1964 to direct the scientists and CSIR labs to actively take up consultancy with the industry both on a 'personal basis' and 'institutional basis,' which was not a prevalent practice till then (Report of the Third Reviewing Committee of Scientific and Industrial Research, 1965). Even after this recommendation, the contribution of government-funded laboratories to industrial output was less than 1% in the late 1970s and early 1980s (Alam & Langrish, 1985). Even the results of technology licencing through NRDC were not satisfactory. For instance, till 1973, of a total of 1,125 technologies reported by CSIR to NRDC, only 446 were licenced to the industry (DST, 1974).

CSIR was involved in performing both basic and applied research in equal proportions. However, given the disappointing performance of CSIR with respect to increasing productivity, it was "dictated" to cut its investments in basic research to 20% (Sandhya, Jain, & Mathur, 1990). CSIR was literally forced to only conduct time-bound R&D which could ensure results useful to increase the productivity of the industry. The Planning Commission during the fourth plan period withheld the CSIR plan proposals and "insisted on submission of proposals project-wise and on a priority" (ibid., p. 2802). Much of the growth of PFRLs like CSIR in India took place at the cost of the universities. Given the concerns of self-reliance and ambitious productivity goals, resources were diverted away from universities and towards PFRLs (Maiti, 2013; Raina, 2006; Krishna, 2001). This move of neglecting universities was heavily criticised by Meghanad Saha, the noted physicist in the country, and even Homi Bhabha, who was one of the crucial persons in the making of India's science policy and a close aide of the country's first PM Jawaharlal Nehru (Krishna, 2001). The most important touchdown in CSIR's history took place when its sixth review committee—famously known as the Abid Hussain Committee—in 1986, mandated that CSIR generate 33% of its revenues on its own (Singh, 1987).

IISc and IITs

IISc is one university in India which was into the process of commercialisation right from its inception. In fact, the idea behind the establishment of IISc by Jamsetji Tata[1] was to have an institution that could help in his business endeavours close to home. The institute was established in 1909 jointly with Tata, colonial GoI, and the Mysore Maharajas.[2] Tata envisaged that the institute should work "in particular, in such branches of knowledge as are likely to promote material and industrial welfare of India" (IISc, 2019). After Independence, IISc was made into a public institute fully funded by the state with the status of a deemed to be university. IISc involves itself with private industry in numerous ways. It used to receive a lot of philanthropic donations and endowment funds right from the beginning, which still continues. Other forms of interaction that took place with the industry during this period and which still continues are sponsored research projects, consultancy with the industry and the establishment of industry chairs. The initial interaction with private industry in IISc took place through individual and informal contacts of the faculty members. This was later institutionalised in 1975 through the establishment of the Centre for Scientific and Industrial Consultancy (ibid.). There is a dearth of details that are available in the public domain about the nature of these interactions. A former professor of IISc who went on to become the director of the institute went on to say the following about such interactions:

> Here, interactions with industry have traditionally been through individual arrangements with faculty. But the situation is rapidly changing with major multinational corporations have begun to make efforts to enter into

wide ranging "collaborations." New models have come into existence, where even research laboratories of companies have entered campuses, in a manner reminiscent of arrangements in the West. These happenings have brought in their wake many problems that need to be addressed. Very often, the memoranda of understanding (MoU) signed between the academic and industrial partners are shrouded in secrecy. The lack of transparency fuels speculation on the nature of arrangements; the general impression is that academic institutions negotiate from a position of weakness, resulting in agreements that are loaded in favour of the industrial partner.

(Editorial, 1999)

The case of IITs was also more or less similar, with sponsored research and industry-funded chairs and research laboratories. There are currently 20 IITs, and all the IITs have established separate organisations to handle such relationships with the industry. It suffices to say here that IITs were into the business of commercialisation similar to IISc right from their inception in the early 1950s (Khokhar & Tewari, 2017).

Liberalisation and the Conquest of Innovation Period

In 1991, India liberalised its economy and opened its markets, allowing foreign capital to operate in the country. It was during this period that the global economy was also moving towards what is called a knowledge econ-omy. Additionally, as a part of the WTO TRIPS Agreement, countries like India were obliged to transform their IPR policies. Till then, the IPR policy, the Indian Patent Act 1970, implemented in 1972, allowed only for process patents for a period of five years in important sectors such as pharmaceu-ticals. With the signing of the TRIPS Agreement, the Patent Act, 1970, was amended in 1995 with a window period of ten years for its implementa-tion. From 2005, implementing the TRIPS Agreement, the patent regime in India got transformed from process patents to product patents. In such an economic landscape, universities and research organisations were under-going a transformation in order to respond to the upcoming challenges. The major characteristics of this transformation were new forms of inter-action with the private industry and the establishment of new institutions for the commercialisation of knowledge and normalisation of such a pro-cess. These new forms of interaction were unlike the previous forms which were demand driven in nature. In the previous forms of interaction, the engagement of the university with private industry was only in the form of consultancy and sponsored research projects and in a few instances estab-lishing laboratories that were of direct value to the private partners. The current forms of interaction are significantly different from the previous forms, in the sense that *they are reminiscent of the characteristics of the neoliberal supply-side logic.* In this scenario, the universities and academic institutes are to do commercially viable R&D irrespective of the existence of any direct demand. The scientists are to carry out their research *'work'* to keep *'supply'* in abundance despite there being no demand at the current moment. This is evident from the tendency to overemphasise the need to generate IP that is *'expected'* to generate economic returns. In order to carry out this new mission, several new entities such as TTOs with management professionals, scientific entrepreneurs where regular faculties and academic institutes were allowed to establish start-ups with an equity stake, and TBIs came into existence. The supply-side-oriented reform processes took place in an incremental manner. They were first implemented in CSIR laboratories, encompassing all of the academia with time.

The Planning Commission of India (2006) appointed a Working Group on Strengthening Academia-Industry Interface (including PPP) with Prof. R. A. Mashelkar[3] as its chairperson. Of the five recommendations provided by the group, one reads "promote movement of technology from laboratory to market place through technology transfer and new venture creation" (ibid., p. 5). As a part of this recommendation, it was suggested that there was a necessity to increase the number of research parks and TBIs close to academic centres. It was also recommended as part of the supply-side incentives that the "government should make land available adjacent to these institutions and provide the highest possible concessions like all benefits of SEZ,[4] concession in electricity tariffs, duty exemption for imported equipment etc" (ibid., p. 9). Recommendations were also made to increase high-technology start-ups by the creation of VCs. The report further noted that the prevailing provisions do not give freedom to scientists to set up commercial entities while in professional employment with universities and institutions and recommend the government evolve facilitating provisions in service rules. Following this, in 2009, GoI issued a memorandum titled "Encouraging Development and Commercialisation of Inventions and Innovations: A New Impetus" (CSIR, 2009) to all the PFRLs and universities. The key initiatives that were put in place through this memorandum are

a.   permitting the researchers to have an equity stake in scientific enterprises/spin-offs while in professional employment with their research and academic organisations,
b.   permitting the scientific establishment to invest in the knowledge base as equity in enterprises,
c.   encouraging scientific establishments to set up incubation centres, and
d.   facilitating the mobility of researchers between industry and the scientific establishment.

The rationale provided for these initiatives was that they would ensure economic growth. The initiatives were also taken with an intent not just to commercialise the knowledge base but also to 'unleash' the entrepreneur in the scientist, which can contribute to economic growth. The document talks about the Massachusetts Institute of Technology, University of Cambridge, and Stanford University; provides their trajectories as evidence; and concludes that such initiatives are inevitable and the only way. And also to reduce the impediments that come along with rising investments for the knowledge-based companies and start-ups, the initiative of knowledge equity was introduced. Under this initiative, the scientific establishments could exchange their knowledge base with the enterprises for an equity stake.

The next important initiative was the establishment of TBIs at academic institutes to provide resources to start-ups and also help them through hand-holding mechanisms with the expertise available at these establishments. The associated academic institute was called the host institute, which provided support services, such as the infrastructure that was present in the laboratories of these scientific establishments at a subsidised cost, and this cost could also be exchanged in the form of equity. Currently, there are around 140 publicly funded TBIs in the country (Surana, Singh, & Sagar, 2018). These are supported by funding from various agencies, such as DST, DBT, Ministry of Small and Medium Enterprises, and more recently through schemes such as the Atal Innovation Mission (AIM). Under corporate social responsibility (CSR), big corporations are allowed to donate for the establishment of TBIs (Kalra, 2019), which was previously only restricted to welfare activities. More recently, CSR was also extended to sponsor research projects in universities (*The Hindu*, 2019).

All of the aforementioned initiatives to encourage entrepreneurship are in resonance with the principles and practices of neoliberalism. The act of putting incentives and institutions in place are reminiscent of what Harvey (2005, p. 2) points to: that under neoliberalism it is believed that

> human well-being can best be advanced by liberating individual entrepreneurial freedom and skills with in an institutional framework characterised by strong private property rights, free markets, and free trade. The role of the state is to create and preserve institutional framework appropriate to such practices.

Secondly, the aforementioned initiatives also echo the same supply-side logic pioneered by President Ronald Reagan in the US during his period and what came to be known as Reaganomics. In the macro-economic context, the idea of supply-side economics is conflated with tax incentives and fewer regulations with an expectation that there would be an increase in investment and thereby production and growth. When it comes to a more sectoral level, initiatives like the ones mentioned earlier provide evidence of the concrete measures put in place to ensure the incentivising of the supply-side. As a means of boosting the supply-side, the academic institutions are expected to ensure that there are necessary inputs (in the form of technologies, ideas, or subsidised infrastructure) that can be put to use in production. The following sections will provide details of how the supply-side mechanisms were implemented at the institutional level, such as CSIR, IISc, IITs, and universities.

To sum up, the new forms of commercialisation that became dominant in the supply-side regime are

a.   technology transfer through patents co-ordinated by TTOs,
b.   scientific entrepreneurs and knowledge equity, and
c.   TBIs.

This is not to say that the previous modes of interaction are absent and are replaced by these new modes of knowledge commercialisation. The argument here is that the forms of knowledge commercialisation which were dominant previously (demand driven) also exist with these new initiatives, but the focus of the scientific establishments in the contemporary economic landscape is more driven towards these new forms of commercialisation. The following sections will provide details of how the supply-side ideas influenced the organisation of knowledge production in academic spaces, such as CSIR, DBT autonomous institutes, IISc, IITs, and central universities.

CSIR

CSIR was the first mover responding to the changes in the nature of the economy (Gupta, Bhojwani, & Koshal, 2000; Krishna, 2007). The kind of transformation that CSIR went through can be understood by two statements given as a call to the scientists by then director general of CSIR Prof. Ramesh Mashelkar. He gave a call that CSIR, which is known as Council for Scientific *and* Industrial Research, should transform itself into the Council for Scientific Industrial Research (Sunder Rajan, 2002). He also stated that the earlier vision of scientists—i.e. 'publish or perish'— should be replaced with 'patent or perish' (*Nature*, 2006). The changes are also a result of the initiatives that were put in place after Abid Hussain's committee recommendations that CSIR should venture into the paradigm of self-financing its research by generating at least 33% of its finances. During this period, CSIR received an interest-free loan from the WB under its Industrial Technology Development Programme 1990. Under this scheme, four CSIR laboratories received a loan amount of 13 million USD (Mashelkar, 2004). Of this, the National Chemical Laboratory (NCL), Pune, had received a loan amount of 5.5 million USD. This loan amount was used by NCL to upgrade its infrastructure, and during this period, it was able to negotiate a successful technology transfer agreement with General Electric, one of the biggest multinational conglomerates based in the US (NCL, 2019). The director of NCL during this success story was Prof. Mashelkar. Given this success, a "Committee on Commercialisation of CSIR Knowledge Base" was appointed under his leadership by GoI to provide a trajectory for the CSIR labs to follow in order to emulate similar success. The result of the committee is a document titled "CSIR Vision and Strategy 2001." In 1995–96, Prof. Mashelkar was appointed as the director general of CSIR, and the recommendations of the aforementioned committee were put in practice. The striking feature of this document is that it explicitly provides evidence of the new forms of commercialisation and corporatisation of knowledge production. It characterises R&D as a *'business activity'* and scientists as *'knowledge workers'* and *'entrepreneurs.'* The case of CSIR is also important because it was the so-called successful trajectory of CSIR that was considered a blueprint for others to follow in the country.

The vision document (1996) set forward several goals to be achieved by 2001. They are

a. to self-finance by generating over seven billion rupees[5] (Indian) from external sources of which at least 50% from the industry. During 1994–95, CSIR was earning 1.35 billion rupees out of which 15% was from industrial source; and

b. to hold a patent bank of 500 foreign patents (up from 50), generate 10% of operational expenditure from licencing and 40 million (US) dollars from contract research service to overseas companies.

The document also laid down a strategic road map to achieve these objectives. It called for restructuring of its organisation to compete in the "global knowledge marketplace" (CSIR, 1996, p. 7). The new strategy envisages CSIR as a corporate entity and each of its labs as a "subsidiary corporate entity" (ibid.). The director of each institute would be the 'CEO' (chief executive officer) assisted by an executive council. A new mechanism of granting autonomy based on the performance of each laboratory in terms of the goals mentioned earlier was also proposed. "[T]he higher the growth rate committed and achieved, higher will be the level of independence from HQs [headquarters], and the laboratory rewarded suitably" (ibid., p. 7).

Further, the document goes on to say that there is no alternative for CSIR but to view R&D as a business and directs each laboratory to evolve a five-year business plan. It calls for shedding the research that cannot optimise economic returns on investment. Also, an effective marketing system is strategised where "the entrepreneur in a scientist would be wakened, equipped and motivated to venture out in the knowledge market space" (ibid., p. 4).

CSIR had a patent office right from its beginning. However, the office was dysfunctional given the general patent scenario in the country. It was only with the vision document and the success of NCL that patents became a prominent part of the scientific life at CSIR. In terms of patents, the vision document advocated that CSIR should file over 1,000 patents every year, with 500 foreign patents. The earlier policy of sharing royalties with scientists which was revoked due to the dismal performance of CSIR with respect to industrial activity was again reintroduced, and 40% of the royalty income was to go to the scientists and 60% to the respective labs (ibid.). Table 4.2 provides the number of patents filed by CSIR from 1995 to 2002.

Table 4.2 Patents Filed by CSIR between 1995 and 2002

S. No	Year	Patents Filed	
		Indian	Foreign
1.	1995–96	260	58
2.	1996–97	209	71
3.	1997–98	264	91
4.	1998–99	310	112
5.	1999–2000	248	199
6.	2000–01	409	450
7.	2001–02	413	580

Source: Gupta (2015).

It can be seen from Table 4.2 that during 1995–96, CSIR filed only for 58 foreign patents, which went up to 580 by 2002. While there is no discrete year-wise data that is available with regard to the number of patents that were granted, a study by Abrol (2007) cites that during the period that is envisaged, CSIR was granted a total number of 591 Indian patents and 101 foreign patents, with only 4% of patents in force licenced. Another important detail that this study gives is that during the aforementioned period, CSIR's division of the Societal and Technological Mission that was addressing the issues of social concern and rural development was dismantled.

Going beyond 2002, Table 4.3 provides details about the number of Indian and foreign patents filed, granted, and licenced. The numbers indicate an increased and vigorous patenting by CSIR. It can be witnessed how the intensity measured in terms of patents filed has escalated over time.

While a direct correlation between the number of patents filed, granted, and licenced in a given year may be misleading, these numbers, when looked at holistically, indicate how supply-side promotion championed by neoliberal economics fares in actuality. Between 1996 and 2018, CSIR filed a total of more than 16,000 patents, of which only 7% were licenced (Viswajanani, 2019). The disproportionality in terms of the number of patents licenced and the number of patents filed is an indicator of how there is an *oversupply in anticipation of the arising of demand* in line with the supply-side logic propounded by neoliberal theory.

Not that this aggressive patenting comes without any cost. To file and maintain patents is in itself an expensive and legally fraught process. In response to an appeal under the Right to Information (RTI) Act, 2005, filed by one Prasad Reddy in 2012, CSIR disclosed that it spent Rs 742.4 million just to file patents. A whopping 97% of this money was spent on filing patents outside of India (Reddy, 2012). According to Dr. Girish Sahni, the former director general of CSIR, it costs Rs 0.2 million to file an Indian patent and more than 20,000 USD for a US patent. Not that this attitude of CSIR was not criticised. In a news item titled "Is India's Patent Factory Squandering

Table 4.3 Patents Filed, Granted, and Licenced by CSIR between 2000 and 2019

S.no	Year	Patents Filed		Patents Granted		Patents Licenced
		Indian	Foreign	Indian	Foreign	
1.	2000–01	409	452	117	62	–
2.	2001–02	413	580	342	94	4
3.	2002–03	421	728	166	191	35
4.	2003–04	406	495	275	218	50
5.	2004–05	418	500	175	272	58
6.	2005–06	407	570	276	179	53
7.	2006–07	169	655	169	316	57
8.	2007–08	207	256	395	331	26
9.	2008–09	183	404	703	333	68
10.	2009–10	161	179	145	319	47
11.	2010–11	174	220	260	361	30
12.	2011–12	NA	NA	NA	NA	26
13.	2012–13	199	436	108	278	NA
14.	2013–14	265	449	92	382	NA
15.	2014–15	310	485	65	339	NA
16.	2015–16	324	523	115	329	NA
17.	2016–17	225	333	101	331	NA
18.	2017–18	170	199	171	371	NA
19.	2018–19	208	174	167	271	NA

Source: (Ajay & Sangamwar, 2014; Viswajanani, 2019).
NA—Not available

Funds?" that appeared in *Nature* (2006), Mashelkar was criticised for turning CSIR labs into "patent factories." Given such increasing expenditure, recently, CSIR labs were mandated that 25% of expenses for the prosecution and maintenance of Indian patents and 50% for foreign patents should be borne by themselves (*Times of India*, 2016). Also, CSIR was always reluctant in disclosing its royalties despite the fact that it is a publicly funded body and is obliged to do so (Reddy, 2012). The mission of self-financing that led to its corporatisation in 1996 is still not complete, and more recently in 2015, the GoI issued a statement directing CSIR labs to increase their external revenues with "ground breaking technologies" (*Nature*, 2018). Overall, till now, the trajectory can be simply put as follows. The self-financing paradigm encouraged patenting and given that patents could not ensure desirable results, the labs are now obligated to generate their own resources to even patent.

The other forms of neoliberal measures other than the oversupply of patents are the emergence of TBIs and scientific entrepreneurs. Immediately after the issuing of the memorandum by the GoI in May 2009, CSIR passed an order on 30 November 2009 implementing the policy. It has established several institutions and TBIs as a means to implement the policy (CSIR, 2009).

One of the institutions established for this purpose was CSIR-Tech Private Limited to make easy the process of establishing spin-offs by CSIR scientists. Currently, CSIR has 12 spin-offs (Viswajanani, 2019) and aims to make it 50 by 2022 (CSIR, 2011). Coming to the case of TBIs, currently, 15 CSIR laboratories are hosting TBIs, and it has made plans to have a TBI in each of its laboratories, and for this purpose, in 2016, it initiated a fund called the CSIR Innovation Fund with Rs 400 billion (CSIR, 2016). Of the TBIs currently existing, Venture Centre, hosted by NCL, is the oldest one, established in 2007. Start-ups incubated at Venture Centre have access to the resources in the form of expensive technological infrastructure, seed grants from various government organisations, patent facilitation centres, and a huge pool of scientific talent. Given the enactment of GoI that academic institutions can participate in commercial ventures through knowledge equity, a large number of start-ups associated with Venture Centre are based on such transactions in the name of the Venture Centre Incubatee Partnership Scheme (Venture Center, n.d.).

IISc

IISc had a similar trajectory as CSIR during this period. It also established various institutions to encourage the commercialisation of knowledge through patenting, as well as through scientific entrepreneurs and TBIs. IISc had a TBI even before CSIR laboratories. The name of IISc's TBI is the Society for Innovation and Development (SID), established in the year 1991. The organisation that takes up patenting and technology licencing is the Intellectual Property and Technology Licensing (IPTeL) office. Initially, IPTel was called the Intellectual Property Cell when established in 2004 and later renamed IPTel in 2015. IPTel provides different pictorial representations of the number of patents filed and granted to IISc over the last two decades. The data from these representations provide evidence similar to CSIR, which is the disproportionate ratio between the number of patents licenced and filed (Table 4.4).

Between 1996 and 2016, IISc filed a total of 717 patents, of which 455 were filed with the Indian Patent Office and the remaining 262 at foreign patent offices (see Table 4.5). Of the 717 patents it filed, it was granted nearly 20%, amounting to 151 (IISc, 2018). One can understand from these numbers the disproportionate ratio between the number of patents granted and filed. This disproportionality only increases if one looks at the ratio of the number of patents licenced and filed. A total of 45 patents were licenced between 1996 and 2016 by the IISc, which is just 6.27% of the total patents filed. The ratio of patents licenced to the number of patents filed shows a similar picture as CSIR, with an oversupply of patents.

There was an attempt to find out the details of the licenced patents and the forms in which they were licenced (exclusive/non-exclusive) under the RTI.[6] However, IISc did not disclose these details. The institute responded to the RTI, saying that the information was not available in the office. It is

Table 4.4 Patents Filed by IISc

S. NO	Year	Patents Filed in	
		Indian	Foreign
1.	1996	2	–
2.	1997	2	–
3.	1998	6	–
4.	1999	12	–
5.	2000	8	6
6.	2001	12	4
7.	2002	11	5
8.	2003	14	12
9.	2004	20	10
10.	2005	14	7
11.	2006	15	18
12.	2007	16	10
13.	2008	33	41
14.	2009	40	35
15.	2010	22	5
16.	2011	39	30
17.	2012	43	42
18.	2013	24	10
19.	2014	39	10
20.	2015	44	12
21.	2016	39	5
22.	**Total**	455	262

Source: IISc (2018).

ironic that despite having a separate organisation to handle IP-related issues, the institute declared that it has no information available. Not to forget the importance of licencing in the whole IP scenario. However, the RTI application disclosed that the revenue-sharing agreement between the scientist and institute in the case of a licenced patent is in the ratio of 60:40.

Coming to the case of scientific entrepreneurs, IISc is the first academic space in India that has rolled out a spin-off[7] by one of its faculty members through SID. All the faculty members of IISc who would like to start a commercial venture are associated with SID. SID also hosts other start-ups. Till 2016, from IISc, seven spin-offs had been rolled out (Pulakkat, 2015). The equity sharing of IISc with the start-ups it hosts for the exchange of services is between 5% and 15%, and the IP to these start-ups is licenced free of cost with an agreement that 1% of product sales are shared as royalty (Ramakrishnan, 2016).

IITs

IITs also pose a similar kind of performance with regard to patents and entrepreneurship. All the IITs have a dedicated TTO for the management of IP and technology transfers. Between 2010 and 2015, the first-generation IITs filed

Table 4.5 Details of First-Generation IITs between 2010 and 2015*

S. No	Name of the IIT	Patents		Technology Transfers	TTO/ Incubator	Number of Incubates	Number of Start-Ups
		Filed	Granted				
1.	Bombay	439	61	73	Yes	71	>26
2.	Madras	311	24	22	Yes	95	89
3.	Delhi	146	25	16	Yes	44	16
4.	Kharagpur	231	13	11	Yes	172	104
5.	Kanpur	204	9	56	Yes	52	26
6.	Guwahati	61	6	5	Yes	13	10

Source: Khokhar & Tewari (2017).
* Data with regard to the number of patents filed and granted till 2019 is available at https://www.iitsystem.ac.in/?q=patents/publicview&year=2019–2020. However, details with regard to technology transfer and the number of start-ups are not available.

Table 4.6 Details of Second-Generation (Established before 2000) IITs

S. No	Name of the IIT	Patents		Technology Transfers	TTO/ Incubators
		Applied	Granted		
1.	Roorkee	22	3	0	Yes
2.	Bhubaneswar	10	0	0	Yes
3.	Gandhi Nagar	4	0	0	Yes
4.	Patna	9	0	0	Yes
5.	Jodhpur	5	0	0	Yes
6.	Ropar	>10	0	0	Yes
7.	Indore	7	0	0	Yes
8.	Mandi	1	0	0	Yes
9.	Varanasi	9	3	0	Yes
10.	Hyderabad*	26	2	NA	Yes

Source: Khokhar & Tewari (2017).
* Includes only Indian patents.

for nearly 1,500 patents and were granted 138 patents, which was less than 10%. The total number of technologies licenced during this period was 185, which was 12.33% of the total patents sought. TBIs were also present in 20 IITs to promote entrepreneurship. Tables 4.5 and 4.6 provide comprehensive details with regard to patents, TTOs, incubators, and the number of start-ups.

However, this kind of rigorous patenting phenomenon in IITs also started after 1995, which is the year of the introduction of the product patent regime. For example, IIT Delhi, one of the oldest IITs, filed only 15 patent applications between 1963 and 1995 (Khokhar and Tewari, 2017). In 1995, after the establishment of its IPR unit, more than 200 applications were filed (ibid.). In fact, in the year 2019, IIT Delhi filed over 150 patents, registering a 20% increase in comparison to the previous year (IIT Delhi, 2019).

DBT Institutes

From the year of its inception, DBT has been instrumental in establishing research institutes and university-level departments. Currently, there are over 15 autonomous research institutions under DBT. These institutes conduct R&D and act as a strong linkage in a step towards commercialising the research results through patents and licencing them. All of these institutes, in their objectives, specify their role in promoting the industry by embedding themselves in the value chain at the level of R&D, providing instrumentation facilities and technology transfers. DBT established an institution named the Biotechnology Patent Facilitation Cell in 1994 to provide assistance to all biologists and biotechnologists in India. It has also taken the initiative to establish multi-institutional regional clusters to ensure connectivity between different institutions and stakeholders in the cluster region (DBT, Pioneering Biotech Innovation, 2016).

In addition to a central patenting cell at the DBT, all the autonomous institutions have their own TTOs. A few institutions even host TBIs, and the scientific entrepreneurship scheme is also encouraged by DBT. An RTI was filed with DBT and its autonomous institutes to provide information with regard to the number of patents filed, licenced, royalties earned, and spin-offs from each institute. Of the 15 institutes, 12 institutes responded to these questions. Again, the evidence from these institutes is also a clear indication of the oversupply of patenting and an abysmal number of licencing deals. DBT institutes in comparison to CSIR and IISc have a very low number of patents granted. Table 4.7 provides details of the patent scenario in each of the DBT institutes.

It was with the establishment of DBT that biotechnology in India found a new impetus. The academic institutes that DBT established have an equal focus if not less on the commercial prospects of their research. This can be understood from the fact that more than half of the institutes mentioned in Table 4.7 host TBIs on their campuses. Each of these institutions also has its own TTOs in order to ensure that the research being carried out is patentable and to find out potential partners to licence it. The data in terms of number of patents filed, granted and licenced also testifies to how there is an oversupply of technologies.

According to DBT, in total, it has 155 patents both from the Indian Patent Office and foreign patent offices in the last four years (2015 onwards) from all its autonomous institutes, extramural research projects, and public-sector industries. But if one looks at the total number of patents filed, it is 406 (DBT, n.d.). And it is very much possible that the foreign patents filed with a single application through the Patent Cooperation Treaty (PCT)

Table 4.7 Patent, TBI, and Spin-Off Data of DBT Autonomous Institutes

S. No	Name of the Institute	Patents Filed		Granted		Licenced	Royalties (in Rs)	Spin-Offs	TBIs
		Indian	Foreign	Indian	Foreign				
1.	Centre for DNA Finger Printing and Diagnostics	8	4	2	6[8]	0	0	0	0
2.	Institute for Life Sciences	22	2	5	4	1	Yet to be realised	0	Coming up
3.	Institute for Stem Cell Research	3	4	-	-	0	0	1 (in process)	Yes
4.	National Centre for Cell Science	24	33	5	17	0	0	0	Associated with Venture Centre (CSIR)
5.	National Agri-Food Biotechnology Institute (NABI)	12	0	In process	0	**	1,353,215	1	Yes
6.	National Institute of Plant Genomic Research	20	31	1	19	3	1,804,000	0	No

7.	National Brain Research Centre	14	19	NA	NA	NA	NA	NA	NA
8.	National Institute of Immunology	NA	NA	12	19	12	16,246,260	0	No
9.	National Institute of Biomedical Genomics	0	0	0	0	0	0	0	No
10.	Regional Centre for Biotechnology	4	0	0	0	0	0	0	Yes
11.	Rajiv Gandhi Centre for Biotechnology	NA	NA	9	6	2	Yet to be realised	NA	Yes
12.	Transnational Health Research Institute	31	24	9	3	5	33,000+ two non-cash transactions	3	Yes

Source: Researcher's compilation through RTIs.

Table 4.8 Year-Wise Number of Patents Granted to Universities[9] in India

S. No	Year	Number of Published[10] Patents	Number of Patents Granted
I	1995	I	I
2	1996	0	0
3	1997	0	2
4	1998	2	3
5	1999	5	4
6	2000	5	6
7	2001	5	5
8	2002	6	8
9	2003	20	24
10	2004	24	25
11	2005	47	21
12	2006	47	33
13	2007	56	33
14	2008	66	25
15	2009	138	33
16	2010	112	33
17	2011	193	20
18	2012	284	26
19	2013	270	9
20	2014	273	3
21	2015	410	7
22	2016	486	2
23	2017	848	I
24	2018	402	0
25	2019	125	-

Source: https://ipindiaservices.gov.in/PublicSearch/PublicationSearch/PatentSearchResult, n.d.

mechanism can lead to multiple grants. From Table 4.8, it can also be seen how abysmally low the numbers of licencing agreements are. Among the 12 institutions mentioned in Table 4.7, licencing deals are available for ten institutes. All ten institutes were able to licence merely 23 patents and filed applications for 255 patents of which 120 were granted. One has to keep in mind that in these 23 licencing deals, there is a possibility that one technology can be a part of more than one licencing deal. For example, the National Agri-Food Biotechnology Institute has filed for 12 Indian patents, and none of them have been granted as of now, but still, it had a licencing agreement with ten entities, all in non-exclusive form, and earned a total royalty of Rs 1,353,215.

If one juxtaposes the cases of CSIR laboratories, IISc, IITs, and DBT institutes, the following similarities emerge:

a. All of these institutions have mechanisms in place to promote the neo-liberal supply-side market logic.

b. There is an oversupply of patents which is disproportionately higher than the number of licencing deals, providing evidence of the supply-side logic propounded by the theory of neoliberalism.

In the following section, the case of Indian universities is explicated to explain how corporatisation took place.

Universities

Unlike PFRLs, universities were not very prominently involved in interacting with private industry, although there was no formal restriction placed on them. However, it was expected that with liberalisation and amendments to the patent law, there would be a shift in the practices of the university. Between 1990 and 2002, excluding IITs and IISc, the patents granted to universities in India were very low in number. According to a study (Bhattacharya, 2005) commissioned by the Principal Scientific Advisor, GoI, which considered institutes like IITs and IISc also as universities, reported that between 1990 and 1994, three universities participated in patenting, between 1994 and 1998 eight universities, and between 1999 and 2002 21 universities participated in patenting. The total number of patents granted during this period to universities was 173. Of these 173, IITs and IISc together had 99 patents, and even among the remaining 74, 41 patents were granted to just one university (ibid.). So, between 1990 and 2002, the number of patents granted virtually to all the Indian universities is just 33 Indian patents. After 2002, several initiatives and policies were put forth by the GoI to ensure that universities actively participate in the commercialisation process. In 2003, GoI brought out its second science policy post-Independence titled Science & Technology Policy 2003, which directed the universities to establish TTOs as associate organisations to the universities (Bhattacharya & Arora, 2007). Thereafter, incremental reforms were witnessed with an active state role, leading to increased commercial activity by the universities. In 2005, GoI appointed the National Knowledge Commission (NKC), which recommended a legal framework to "revitalise research in universities and give an impetus to publicly funded research" by providing universities and research institutions ownership of their inventions arising out of state funding (GoI, 2009). This recommendation is similar to the Bayh-Dole Act enacted in the US that led to the commercialisation of publicly funded research.

In India, currently, there are 911 universities of which nearly 600 are publicly funded (UGC, 2019). In the last two decades, all of the universities together have filed for a total number of 3,840—a massive increase from just 33—Indian patents of which more than 90% of filings took place only after 2008. We can see from Table 4.8 how these reforms have led to this increase in patent filings by Indian universities.

While licencing data of all universities together is not available, a scant amount of data for the years 2012–13, 2013–14, and 2014–15 is available for select universities in the form of a National Institution Ranking Framework (NIRF) report. According to these reports, major central universities like Jawaharlal Nehru University, Delhi University, and the University of Hyderabad didn't licence any patents during this period.

Further, to encourage incubators and entrepreneurship in the universities, the GoI's memo of 2009 "Encouraging Development and Commercialisation of Inventions and Innovations: A New Impetus" was also made applicable to universities. The decade starting from 2010 was declared as a decade of innovation and the GoI appointed the National Innovation Council (NIC) as an implementing agency towards this goal. The council suggested the creation of cluster innovation centres in universities based on the experience of countries like the US (Office of Adviser to the Prime Minister, 2011). The council suggested a list of several functions to these clusters of which promotion of entrepreneurship stands first. The functions also include IP portfolio management, technology transfer, and collaboration with the industry. The recommendation of this reform marked the beginning of the evaluation of the performance of universities based on commercial parameters. The parameters are as follows:

a. Patents: applied for and granted
b. Research publications
c. University spin-offs
d. Businesses incubated and success rate
e. Average year-on-year growth of incubated start-ups
f. Revenue generated through technology licencing
g. Curriculum innovation activities
h. Recognitions and awards received

In 2015, University Grants Commission (UGC), the nodal body that governs all the universities in India issued guidelines titled "University-Industry Inter-Linkage Centres in Universities." One of the objectives of this scheme was to help set up TBIs across all universities in India. These centres were planned to be set up in universities with the partnership of an industry. The terms of the partnership were such that the UGC would contribute a maximum of 75% of the expenditure needed to set up the centre, and the industry partner would contribute a minimum of 25% (UGC, 2015). With these initiatives in place, several universities have established TBIs in the recent past. While the emergence of entrepreneurial characteristics in universities lagged behind the PFRLs, none the less they are picking up the pace. The universities also provide evidence of the disproportionate ratio of patents licenced, granted, and filed, vindicating the same supply-side logic witnessed in the case of CSIR laboratories, DBT institutes, IISc, and IITs.

Innovation 2.0—The Coercive Innovation Period

In the earlier period, though policies were put in place to ensure supply-side measures, there was no coercion to implement these policies. But since 2015, universities and academic institutes have been obligated to participate in this process by coercion and through the use of state power, where funding to these universities is linked to the parameters which are of direct relevance towards the corporatisation of universities. 'Naming and shaming' measures are also used as a part of normalising this process. This is in direct contradiction with the autonomy that the public universities were granted, as well as the long-cherished idea of autonomous science.

To put it more concretely, in the year 2015, GoI announced AIM[11] to further enhance the entrepreneurial process and with an expectation that entrepreneurship and innovation would ensure growth and employment. To meet this need, a scheme called Self Employed and Talent Utilization was devised, which is a techno-financial, incubation, and facilitation programme (NITI Aayog, 2015). As a part of this scheme, the GoI was suggested by the NITI Aayog[12] to strengthen the IPR regime in India. In accordance with this recommendation, GoI introduced a new IPR policy in 2016. The new IPR policy mandates all the publicly funded scientists and professors to compulsorily convert all their discoveries into IP assets and predicates their promotions based on the number of patents they secure (Basheer, 2016). The NIRF of the GoI, which assesses the universities and academic institutions for their performance, has made the number of patents that the university secures and the royalties they earn important parameters in their ranking. Extending the proposal of university innovation clusters put forward by the NIC, in 2018, MHRD introduced a scheme termed the Institutional Innovation Council (IIC). The government mandated the universities to set up IICs in all academic centres in the country and as per the government's claim, currently, there are more than 1,000 IICs. The major focus of these IICs are as follows (MHRD[b], 2019):

a. Start-up/entrepreneurship supporting mechanisms in higher educational institutions (HEI)
b. Establish functional ecosystems for scouting ideas and pre-incubation of ideas

These councils are to be constituted with 13 members comprising two technical experts from the nearby industry, two alumni entrepreneurs, one representative from a local TBI, one representative from a leading bank, a patent expert, and three students and faculty members each. The IICs are directed by a central innovation council at MHRD called MHRD's Innovation Cell. The IICs are awarded 'gold stars' (*sic*) based on the implementation of activities mandated by the MHRD. An academic institute can earn a maximum of five gold stars. Another instrument that is being used to evaluate the universities is the Atal Ranking of Institutions on Innovation Achievements (ARIIA). The objective of ARIIA, as stated by the minister of MHRD, is "ARIIA will ensure that innovation is the epicentre of Indian education" (MHRD[a], 2019, p. 8). The following are the parameters used to rank HEIs (ibid.):

a. Budget expenses and revenues generated through innovation and entre-preneurship development—20 'marks'
b. Facilitating access to advanced centres/facilities and entrepreneurial support system—ten 'marks'
c. Idea-to-entrepreneurship data—54 'marks'
d. Development of innovation ecosystem through teaching and learning—ten 'marks'
e. Best innovative solutions developed in-house for improving the governance of an institution—six 'marks'

Universities are evaluated for 100 marks based on the aforementioned parameters, and these rankings are made public on the website specially designed for this purpose (www.ariia.gov.in). These measures are reminiscent of what Kleinman and Vallas (2001) refer to as the industrialisation of academia in their work *Science, Capitalism and the Rise of Knowledge Worker*. If we look at the anatomy of the industrialisation of academia that took place in the US (ibid.), the previously noted policy measures proposed by the GoI are reminiscent of the same. According to Kleinman and Vallas (ibid.), the anatomy of industrialisation of academia in the US comprises five elements and is as follows:

a. Universities and their administration adopt business-like conceptions of academic units.
b. Hiring and promotions are based on quantitative measures, such as external revenues that an individual scientist generates.
c. The influence of IPR and the licencing revenues that are generated by university faculty.
d. Increasing reliance on contract employment and non-standard work arrangement previously only restricted to private industry.
e. Stratification of faculty with respect to the market and market-related activity.

All of these elements can be clearly witnessed in the period which I have term the Coercive Innovation period. The ARIIA framework is exactly this, where the institutions and their scientists are evaluated based on their market-related activity. In 2018, GoI introduced the scheme of graded autonomy (UGC, 2018), similar to the one witnessed in the case of CSIR during the period of its revamp towards more commercial reforms. Graded autonomy simply means that all universities do not enjoy equal autonomy, and the extent of autonomy is determined based on the output of each university. Currently, the output is measured through the National Academic Accreditation score, which considers innovation an important aspect of evaluation. However, looking at the way reforms are progressing, it may not be hard to predict that the autonomy of the university would be more linked to its commercial parameters judged through instruments such as ARIIA.

GoI also brought out another initiative—namely, the National Innovation and Start-Up Policy 2019 for Students and Faculty (MHRD[c], 2019). The policy is to make sure that innovation becomes the epicentre of education, and to meet that need, a guiding framework is provided to universities. The focus of this document is to make sure that the necessary mechanisms are in place to enhance entrepreneurship among students and faculty members. As per the new guidelines, participation in start-up activities is taken into consideration while assessing the faculty members, and it is mandated that universities should ensure that each faculty member mentors at least one start-up. Product development, commercialisation, and nurturing of start-ups are made compulsory for university scientists in addition to teaching and guiding. Universities are allowed to take a stake of 2%–9.5% for the services they provide for the start-ups. The policy document ends by saying, "COMMERCIAL success is the ONLY measure in long run" (ibid., p. 21; emphasis original).

What Do the Scientists in Academia Perceive of This Transformation?

In order to further understand the changes that took place in academia, in-depth interviews were conducted with scientists from a variety of academic institutions across the country. Interviews were conducted with 11 scientists from CSIR, DBT, IIT, ICMR, and central universities to understand how they perceive these changes and also to know about the prevalence of corporate culture and functioning of entities such as TTOs at their respective institutions.

First, in an attempt to understand the historical nature of the interaction between industry and academia, scientists were asked if they have noticed any shift in the nature of the interaction. Most scientists responded that there was always an interaction between the industry and academia in India; however, they say, there is an organised way of interaction with a clear policy focus that is taking place from the last decade because of the liberalisation of Indian economy. The temporal shifts that I have argued in the previous sections become evident from the narrative of this senior scientist from one of the IITs with over 25 years of experience.

This shift has happened ten to fifteen years back. It's not very recent also. Because with the opening of the economy and with the MNCs coming in, the interaction at least between some of the top companies and academia in the country picked up. Now the difference is that there are lots of these startups, and this startup culture increased in the last 4 to 5 years and that is another level of collaboration taking place between public institutions and private money and private capital. But I have been into this system for the last more than twenty-five years. There hasn't been anywhere, anytime, that government has said not to interact.

While I attempted to understand the historical nature of the interaction, scientists were also asked if there is a decline in state funding during the period of increased interaction. In response to this query, almost all the scientists except one opined that the increased interaction is due to a decline in state funding; however, most of them saw it as only one among multiple reasons for the increased interaction with the private industry. It also emerged from the discussion that there is an increasing interest from scientists themselves to interact with the industry:

> People are now aware and want to compete at the world level. So they are looking for an opportunity to interact with the industry to ensure what they are developing will reach the market. So that is the strategy nowadays researchers or scientists are applying.

However, a scientist from ICMR completely dismissed any relationship between state funding and increased interaction with the private industry. She attributed this increased interaction to the change in 'ideology' and the dominance of the knowledge economy. She explained that after the implementation of the product patent regime, there is a need for a symbiotic interaction between industry and academia. Hence there is a 'push-pull' model where there is a push from the government towards innovation, which is then pulled by the industry.

> No. Our philosophy has changed. We were doing the research for the sake of doing research. This [is] a method we adapted long back. Now as we are part of the global knowledge economy, new products are coming which are knowledge based, which are R&D based. So it is very difficult to do the research work in silos either by the industry or by the government. They need some kind of complementation to each other. This is a kind of push and pull model.

Following on, it was further probed, how do the economic benefits in terms of royalties and entrepreneurship prospects such as spin-offs influence scientists? Along with this, it was also probed how the new evaluation system, especially the one pointed out in the previous section "Innovation 2.0—The Coercive Innovation Period" affects them. There were varied responses that came out when this aspect was probed. While some of them perceived that such economic prospects do not have any influence, others noted that it varies from individual to individual. There were also scientists who perceived that economic prospects should in fact influence the scientists so that they get motivated. For instance, a scientist from CSIR expressed this view:

> To a certain extent, yes. It does influence. At least earlier, this question was never asked. Does it have any application? Is this research patentable? Nowadays, it happens regularly. They [scientists] discuss their results with experts and find the commercial angle from that.

Another scientist from an autonomous institute of DBT provided an interesting perspective. He said that gaining economic value out of one's research should be a matter of choice and not be forced:

> So people who want to work on basic research, they want to focus in depth on their own work and not to get distracted by small, small things. Right? For example, if you want a top shot like Virat Kohli kind of effect, you need a discipline, you need a focus and target. He cannot be diluted himself by getting into trivial things. Of course, there are scientists who like to work on [the] translational side also. So they should be encouraged. What I say is, it should not be forced.

Explaining how the current evaluation criteria are replacing the academic value system, this scientist said thus,

> Suppose I can do a very great science, but [what] if my institute's priority is different? They are looking for product development. But I have got an excellent Nature Science paper, but there is no immediate product thing. Now if the evaluation system is geared towards evaluating what the outcome would be, of course those who did great science will fail there. I say there is [a] shift in the valuation system.

The scientist further went on to say how patenting as a system is currently functioning. He said since institutions have made patents an evaluating criterion, even if scientists know that there is very low commercial potential, they end up patenting, spending a lot of money. This scientist felt that such situations are leading to a draining of institutional resources. This is one of the reasons why CSIR has dictated its scientists to earn their own resources to even patent. He also opined that the patenting system poses new kinds of challenges to the scientist, such as worrying about commercial prospects. He further added that with patenting in mind, the scientist has to withhold the research results from publishing, which may sometimes lead to losing the competition with other scientists who might also work in a similar area.

> My personal response is that many people are filing patents, right? So one of the things that has become frequent is "how many patents you

have filed"? There are two types of work which you can patent, right? One thing is show some novelty, commercial potential and patent. But in other cases, you yourself know that commercial potential is weak but still patent (it), spending a lot of money even after knowing that the commercial potential is weak. This happens because institutions have made patenting an evaluating criteria [sic] and instances like these drain an institution's resources only. We are not like big corporations or American universities who have billions of dollars.... But we are not like that. We are a publicly funded organisation and even though we have put a lot of efforts [sic] towards patent and they are not being commercialised, then it becomes a challenge understanding the issue. What should we do? Should we patent or should we forget and do our general things. This is also a distraction for a scientist. Also, the moment you start thinking about patent, you have to withhold your research for some time. You may lose the competition. Suppose if I am working on some project and somebody else in Israel or America is working on the same project. I want to be the first to publish. But the institute says, no, no, let us do patent first and then publish. So essentially his whole work is done but [he] cannot communicate because of this patent business. So he sometimes finds that frustrating. Right? This is the practical problem today. There is no solution right now. Obviously, you have to withhold. If you make it public, you [sic] own work becomes a prior art.

The interviewer also probed whether there was an active TTO in their respective institution and enquired about how it functions and what have been their experiences in interacting with TTOs. All scientists responded that there is a TTO or a similar kind of entity at their respective institutions. For example, the TTO at ICMR is called the IPR unit under the division of innovation and translation. A scientist who was also part of a TTO at one of the DBT's autonomous institutions explained the role of the TTO as a catalyst in linking scientists to the industry.

> While scientists were developing technologies, they lack a catalyst which can link industry and research organisations. TTOs are like a catalyst which fill that space.

A scientist from a CSIR institute, while explaining his interaction with TTO, said that their institution doesn't have a full-fledged TTO, and there is an advisor who advises on the commercial potential of their technology. He said that the advisor also guides the scientists by providing inputs, such as whom to approach and whether the data available is enough to commercialise:

> We do not have full-fledged TTO because we are very small. We have a kind of advisor who looks at the technology and she advises on how

to take it further. We do it on a case-to-case basis. What we do is, once we realise, we discuss with the advisor about the potential of commercialising particular technology. She only advises whom to approach or if we need to generate some more data to be more convincing to the industries to accept our data and she advises how much more data is to be generated. Then we devise mechanisms and money to generate that data. Then she suggests [to] us whom to approach and then we initiate that exercise.

In another CSIR institute, a scientist, while explaining how TTO functions in their institution, said that they conduct some public meetings and workshops to demonstrate the benefits of said technology and identify potential users from those meetings. This is followed by one-on-one meetings where negotiations related to the cost of the technology take place. The scientist explained that there is also a business development team which takes part in these negotiations:

> There are a few stages. We have to do some public meetings and workshops to make people understand what it is. [From such meetings, users are identified.] If user is identified, then there are one-to-one meetings. All paper work is supported by the department. Then cost is negotiated based on what we think of what they can pay and what kind of application and use it will be having. Business development team is also there which will negotiate the deals based on the inputs provided.

Explaining how the TTO functions at ICMR, a scientist was also a part of the IPR unit there said that the IPR unit identifies the leads with commercial potential and files for patents to convert them into "IP assets":

> As a part of the IPR unit, we try to identify the leads which have a more commercial component. Our scientists do both basic and applied research. We try to extract leads from our institute and extra mural projects. We identify the innovative elements there and file patent on it and try to convert this "IP asset" into product.

The terminology that emerged from this particular scientist's response is very interesting and indicates the normalisation of business terminology in academic institutions. This particular scientist, who was a part of a TTO, articulated IP as an "asset." Birch (2017) clearly shows in his work how IP has become an income-deriving asset for all the major stakeholders in the MBT innovation ecosystem, including academia and the fledgling biotech start-ups. The same scientist, on further probing on the process of how leads with commercial potential are identified, revealed that they first start with *sensitising* the scientists about the potential areas in collaboration with business organisations such as FICCI. She explained that such sensitisation has helped scientists in identifying the commercial potential of the technologies they developed. Also, the IPR unit has some template questionnaires through which potential technologies are identified and placed before a committee to make a final decision. She noted,

> First of all, we sensitise our scientists. Recently, we have sensitised our scientists, inviting all of them to a summit or commercialisation programme in association with FICCI. FICCI has given some inputs. After getting sensitised, scientists assessed their research and decided whether they can go ahead with commercialisation. We also interact with scientists through some template questionnaires which have questions like what is the demand? how is it useful? etc. After the filling of questionnaires, we place it before a committee and the committee decides whether or not to go ahead.

Further, when it was enquired whether the TTO advises scientists to keep their information confidential, the same scientist responded by saying, "[S]cientists are smarter than us and we do not give such advice." However, she added that IPR unit also advises scientists to disclose any invention first to them which is followed by an assessment. If the assessment finds the technology patentable, then the IPR unit advises them to file for a 'patent first' and then publish. She noted,

> Actually, scientists are smarter than us. Because this is his/her invention. If a parent whether educated or not educated, know [sic] very well how to keep their baby fit and take care (of it). Inventor is the parent of the invention. They know where to maintain confidentiality. We also sensitise them by asking them to disclose any new invention to the IPR unit first. They report to us, then we advise them about patentability based on assessment which typically takes about 1–2 months. If the invention is patentable, then we advise them to file a patent first and then go for publishing.

In order to further understand the corporatisation of the university, it was enquired whether the TTOs have any employees who have an industrial and marketing background. To this, most scientists responded that their institutions are very small and just setting up TTOs. However, in those institutions where there is a full-fledged TTO, it was clear that there was a remarkable presence of employees from a marketing and industry background.

In the case of ICMR where there is a revamping of the entire technology transfer system, when asked about the presence of marketing staff, they said they are currently outsourcing marketing activities and plan to hire some marketing staff soon. They also said currently, FICCI is supporting them with market assessment. One of the scientists from ICMR noted,

We are outsourcing it to some marketing agencies currently, but we will soon hire someone with a marketing background. We are also taking the help of FICCI. FICCI does market assessment for us.

A director from one of the IITs responded by saying that they try to have people with industrial backgrounds work in the TTO. He explained,

We typically try to have people from an industry background to work in our TTO. In fact, actually in my IIT, the whole industry-academia inter-face is being handled by somebody who was a CEO of Tata Enterprises.

From the previous discussion, it is evident that there is definitely a change in the nature of the interaction between private industry and academia. While there are differences of opinion among the scientists interviewed with regard to such changes and the reasons behind them, none of the scientists have denied this shift. While some have attributed it to the circumstances of the time and the nature of the global economy, others linked it to the open-ing up of the Indian economy and some to the ambitiousness of individual scientists. But what none of them have denied is that there is a new way of interaction between academia and the private industry. It is also clear from the discussion that there is definitely a shift in the value system in the academic environment. We can witness from the scientists' own testimonies about the emergence of new evaluating criteria that are more based on commercial prospects. One scientist also brought out the real-time chal-lenges that scientists face with the advent of the patenting phenomenon. The testimonies from the scientists also confirm the arising of entrepreneur-ial universities with corporate values and culture. The presence of TTOs in all the institutions, their role in the commercialisation process that involves sensitising scientists and the outsourcing work to marketing companies, the involvement of business lobbying organisations like FICCI with scientists, the presence of CEOs who previously helmed big corporate houses all bear testimony to the corporatisation of Indian academia.

Notes

1 The founder of the Tata Enterprises, one of the biggest business conglomerates in India.
2 Rulers of the princely state of Mysore.
3 The discussion of how Prof. R. A. Mashelkar transformed CSIR is described in the subsequent section.
4 Special Economic Zones
5 Currently, one USD is nearly 75 Indian rupees, and this value is determined by the currency markets.
6 The researcher filed the RTIs
7 Details of the spin-off named Strand Genomics were discussed in detail in Chapter 3.

   8 Foreign patents are usually filed using the PCT process in which case an application is counted as one, but the granted patents count can be higher.
   9 Includes all kinds of universities—i.e. public, private, and deemed to be universities.
  10 Every patent application is published before 18 months from the date of receipt of application by the patent office.
  11 Named after former prime minister Atal Bihari Vajpayee.
  12 NITI Aayog replaced the earlier planning commission.

Chapter 5

Production and Accumulation

This chapter discusses the dynamics of production and capital accumulation in the MBT start-ups in India. As a part of such exploration, this chapter specifically examines the organisation of production of the firms in terms of production strategies, employment practices, hierarchy in the organisation, division of labour, inter-firm relationships, and investment practices. Further, the chapter also examines the role of three critical actors discussed in the previous chapters—namely, state, academia, and financial actors—and how each of these play a role at the firm level in MBT start-ups to further the process of accumulation. There are primarily two reasons why start-ups are chosen for this purpose. First, the MBT ecosystem is specifically constituted to encourage entrepreneurship so that it can lead to economic growth. Secondly, this growth is expected to take place in such a way that the start-ups will enable accumulation for a variety of actors in the form of a successful exit strategy.

In *Capital* Volume 1, Marx (1887: 104) explains that in a simple production process in the capitalist system, accumulation takes place in a single layer through the circulation of capital in which commodities are produced and exchanged for money (M-C-M'; where M' >M). But in the start-up ecosystem, particularly in the case of biopharmaceutical start-ups, the accumulation process is double-layered (see Figure 5.1). This can be demonstrated by what is generally considered a successful exit strategy. A successful start-up either scales up its production through an IPO or takes its innovation to a level where it can be out-licenced to other big firms or end in M&A. In the case of out-licencing, accumulation takes place for the start-ups, for the investors in the start-ups, and its employees with stock options, as well as for the firm that licenced it. In the case of M&A, start-ups and their investors get returns on their investment by selling the firm, and the firm that acquires it gets complete rights on the start-up and the products that are developed or in the pipeline and their IP assets. In some cases, acquisitions are also done in order to avoid competition and to secure one's own market. The revenues earned by the start-up both in the form of out-licencing or an M&A are the capital investment by the other big firm, which makes further profits by expanding its market. The same logic also applies

DOI: 10.4324/9781003292104-6

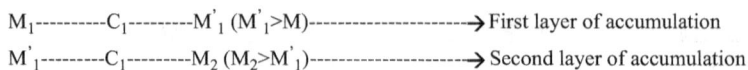

M_1----------C_1---------M'_1 (M'_1>M)---------------------→ First layer of accumulation

M'_1---------C_1---------M_2 (M_2>M'_1)--------------------→ Second layer of accumulation

Where

M_1 is the investment made in the startup

C_1 is the innovation developed by the startup

M'_1 is the profits made through out-license or M&A

However,

M'_1 is also the investment made by the big firm

C_1 is the same innovation licensed or acquired

M_2 is the profit made by the big firm using C_1

Figure 5.1 Double-Layered Accumulation in MBT Start-Ups.

in the case of an IPO where investors exit by diluting their shares and thereby earning their returns and the new investors investing in the start-up. So, unlike in a simple production process where there is a single layer of direct accumulation, the dynamics of accumulation through start-ups is double-layered.

Although in the second process of capital circulation there may be a value addition by the bigger firm, the critical element that determines the market potential is the 'innovation.' Additional capital expenditure for value addition carries its own profit share with the innovation accounting for its own proportion. Hence, the same product/innovation (C_1) leads to a *double-layered accumulation*. This double-layered accumulation is a predominant phenomenon, particularly in the case of innovative biopharmaceutical start-ups.

Second, globally, in the MBT set-up, start-ups came to define the innovative ecosystem and are considered to be central agents of innovation and economic activity. Start-ups are supposed to be risk-taking entities and primarily engage in innovation as an economic activity. Given such a crucial role of start-ups in the innovative process and economic growth, the Indian state aims to have more than 10,000 start-ups specifically in the biotechnology sector by 2024, with an increase of over 270% from the number of biotech start-ups that are currently there (BIRAC[a], 2019). Also, if we look at the first-generation biotech firms discussed in detail in Chapter 1, all of them had a typical start-up trajectory supported by the financial actors, state, and academia. The only difference is that 'start-up' was not a buzzword then, and there was no presence of a stable ecosystem of innovation for MBT. In India, a stable ecosystem started coming up only after NBDS-I, and as mentioned in Chapter 2, by NBDS-II, 'entrepreneurship' became an important focus for DBT, in which start-ups are envisioned to play a major role. Besides, unlike the traditional business set-up, the organisation of economic activity in start-ups is considered to be more flexible and less hierarchical. The relationship between labour and capital in start-ups is considered to be significantly different from an established corporate set-up. So an examination of the start-ups also throws light on an important dynamic of capitalism, which is the relationship between labour and capital.

With this background, the specific questions that are addressed in this chapter are as follows: (a) How is the firm organised? What are the various types of employment practices followed in the MBT start-ups? Who are the various actors that take part in the innovation process of start-ups? (b) What is the role of various actors—namely, financial, state, and academia—in the accumulation strategy of start-ups? (c) What is the exit strategy of MBT start-ups, what is the rationale behind a particular exit strategy, and how does the double-layered accumulation take place?

The chapter mainly draws from in-depth interviews that were conducted with the founders of 20 MBT start-ups from three TBIs in Bengaluru and Hyderabad. Most of the start-ups covered were from the biopharmaceutical sub-sector. Of the 20 start-ups where interviews were conducted, six were in the biopharma sector, five in the medical devices sector, four in medical diagnostics, one in tissue manufacturing, one in enzyme manufacturing, one in CRO, and one in reproductive and regenerative medicine. Of the 20 start-up founders interviewed, seven had previous industry backgrounds, five of them had done their PhDs, three of them had done their postdoctoral research abroad, and the rest had engineering and master's degrees in India. The ages of the firms varied from two to seven years. Most of the founders of medical device firms had an engineering background. The range of issues discussed with the founders included the organisation of the firm, division of labour, salaries, ownership patterns, initial and current sources of capital, relationships with academia and the problems associated with it, relationships or contracts with other firms, role of the state and its institutions, and, finally, exit strategies. The issues of hierarchy and division of labour were also discussed with 14 employees working in these start-ups.

In addition, a case study of a relatively successful biopharmaceutical start-up named Bugworks (BW) is also made in order to further elaborate and put in context all of the previously discussed issues, as well as to further explain how double-layered accumulation takes place.

Process of Production in the MBT Start-Ups

In order to understand the process of production, the founders of start-ups were asked about the number of employees in their firms, the kinds of employment they provide, their salaries and hierarchies in the organisations, inter-firm relationships, and relationships with academia, state, and financial actors. The hierarchy aspect was also examined with the employees of the firm. All of these issues are discussed in detail in the following sections.

Types of Employment and Employment Conditions

The number of employees in the start-ups ranged between two and 12. Most of the employees had finished their education either in life sciences or engineering. Some mature firms also had chartered accountants as their employees. It emerged from the interviews with the founders of the start-ups that they deploy a variety of employment practices, unlike the traditional ones. There were PhD students who were employed in these firms whose research projects are the work they do for these start-ups, employees with stock options, and in several instances, even employees of these firms are provided through government initiatives. While one gets to witness different types of employment practices in these start-ups, it also emerges that these new practices come with their own set of contradictions that are in direct conflict with the interest of employees. For instance, a start-up which is manufacturing technologies for biopharmaceuticals employs PhD students whose salaries are equivalent to the fellowship paid to the PhD students by the GoI in the name of Junior Research Fellowship (JRF). While the founder of the start-up says that by employing PhD students, they are training them to be a part of the labour market by providing them a competitive advantage over the normal PhD students, the firm does not allow these employees to publish their research findings before patenting.

> We don't have employees. We have PhD students who registered with other universities and are working with us in developing technologies. This is something different from other models. We want to raise awareness that PhD students need to be industry experts. Because they shouldn't think that they did a mistake working with academic institutes. I am not saying it is bad, but you don't know what you are really doing except publishing and pursuing your topic. The company works with two principles. Do work and make money. Companies are not doing unnecessary spending, it's something the money is put out from the pocket.

This peculiar practice of equating employment with studentship is further explained by the founder of the firm saying that these students should only work on a particular technology that is of direct economic interest to the firm. Not that these student employees have any extra-economic advantage by engaging in the economic activity of the firm. Student employees are paid a remuneration equivalent to that of a fellowship that a student pursuing a PhD in universities is paid. One of the employers explained,

> Company gives salary to them equal to JRF. They just register with the university and work here in our labs and submit thesis to the university. They are part-time students. They work on a "particular technology only" because we want them to get a patent and paper *in the name of the company*.
> [emphasis added]

Further, explaining how this arrangement of patenting and publishing works and how the work these student employees do is different from the nature of work that is done in universities, the founder of the firm explained as follows:

> First we will file for a provisional patent and then complete the patent and then they can publish. That's the company policy. Because company is *feeding* them, so it should get the benefit out of it. But at the same time, we are helping them to train and once they get out of the PhD, they will be "INDUSTRIALLY TRAINED" (emphasis by the respondent) PhD students. Whereas in academics, in a way they are working with the labs but they may not have any patent. They will move for the postdocs. They don't get industrial options. But these guys can either go for a postdoc or work in the industry.

It also emerged from the interviews with start-up employers that the salaries they provide are usually below the market rates without any social security benefits. For instance, a founder, when asked about the kind of salaries that start-ups provide, explained that while the general trend is to pay below-market rates, he pays a little more, along with providing stock options. However, when this founder revealed the salary he pays, the amount was substantially below the market rate, and even the stock options provided were clouded in a whole lot of terms and conditions.

> My perspective is, startups should pay more than market, because we don't provide health insurance, PF [provident fund] and all that in most cases 99.9%. We have to give more than market. I pay Rs 28,000[1] to one employee. Nobody pays that and stock options.

Further explaining how the system of stock allocation takes place, the same founder detailed that when the employment offer is given, they are also provided with stock options. However, this doesn't mean that the employee gets the promised stock options right from the beginning. The promised stock options are linked to the commitment that these employees provide to the firm in terms of the number of years they work for the firm. The higher the number of years the employee works for the firm, the higher the share allocated, but these shares can only be monetised at the time of exit, which is shredded in high uncertainty.

> Yeah, beginning of the contract, depending on the grade of the entry [about allocation of share]. I have three employees. Two full-time and one part-time. Part-time guy doesn't have any stock option. At the time of giving [the] offer letter, I tell them, so I have a certain ratio, both of them together have slightly less than half. I tell them one-third of the half you will get in a year and one-third next and so on. What does it

mean? It means you have the option to monetise that at the time of the exit. When somebody gives me let's say five-six crores, after two or three or four years, they will get their share.

The situation is even more deplorable in the context of employees provided by the DBT supported public institution Biotechnology Consortium of India Limited (BCIL). BCIL, a public institution supported by DBT, runs a scheme named Industrial Training Programme. While the objective of the programme "is to provide industry-specific training to biotech students for skill development" (BCIL, n.d.), start-ups consider these trainees as employees. This founder who was provided a trainee by the BCIL when asked about the employees in his firm responded as follows:

> One of them is the BCIL candidate. The government will provide *staff* to companies who are in need of manpower. So they will come as a trainee. The government will pay [a] salary to them and also bench fees to the company. So in a way, a student gets Rs 10,000 per month as a salary and the company will get Rs 8,000 in order to train them. These are called BCIL trainees. So it's actually advantageous because they pay the salary.

What emerges when looking at the employment practices is that start-ups are deploying a variety of employment practices unlike the practices in a typical corporate set-up. However, almost all of the start-up founders interviewed reported salaries far below the market rates. Interestingly, all the founders of these firms cast their employment practices as benevolent, such as in the case of employing PhD students where a founder said that these students are advantageous when it comes to labour market competition or a founder who said that he provides stock options to the employees. But as it comes out from their own narrative, the employees are severely restricted in some of most the crucial aspects that are vital for their personal growth. For example, the student employees cannot publish till the innovations are patented, and, typically, a patent takes 18 months even to get published in India and a minimum of three to four years to get awarded. Similarly, the employer who says that he provides stock options attaches several terms and conditions, and these stocks can only be diluted if the start-ups have a successful exit, which itself is highly uncertain.

Another important aspect examined to understand the organisation of the firm is the division of labour and hierarchy in the firm. It is generally believed that start-ups provide a flexible work environment when compared with an established traditional corporate set-up. When enquired about this aspect, almost all the founders responded that theirs is a very small organisation with no hierarchy. However, they explain that there is a division of work among them, but the divisions are not as rigid as in a big corporate firm.

> Absolutely no [hierarchies]. Here everybody knows what we are doing. Everybody is connected. We all interact and from day one, I have been telling like it's our project and there's nothing like one person is going to handle this. All of us work together.

Most of the employees also echoed a similar opinion, although there was a contrasting opinion that emerged. In fact, few employees expressed the view that they chose to work in the start-up because of this absence of a rigid division of labour similar to what Fochler (2016) observed in the case of Austrian biotech start-up employees. Almost all the employees worked between eight to nine hours.

> Great [about the relationship with the employer]. I started my career with this company only. We have been taught that there is a huge difference between boss and employees, [but here] this [is] my table, and my boss sits there. This is our office from where we start[ed] and that's the assembly process. Hardly five feet of the distance he sits. Whatever problems I am facing, I can directly share with him and he is a person who is always here to help you and any time any place. Each and every aspect. I have talked to my friends who work in other firms regarding their work culture. I would say I am very lucky to work here.

From the narratives of the employees, it also emerged that most of them attribute a meaning of learning and skill development to their employment rather than the routine work, in which salaries and perks matter more. Also, the overwork that employees often do was justified as "working for themselves" since they are offered equity (with conditions) and the working environments are kept flat without apparent hierarchies.

> In a startup, one more important thing is that the *hierarchy* is very less. There will be very less employees and you will be directly interacting with the directors. In our case, our directors are very well established with more than 15 years of industrial experience who have worked in good companies like Biocon, Dr. Reddy's. So we gain [a] lot of things out of direct interaction. That's also a plus point.

While most employees echoed a similar opinion to that of their employer with respect to hierarchy and division of labour, this was not a unanimous response. For example, the following employee felt his opinion was not considered in the decision-making process. He also felt that his employer used words like "family" only to extract more work. He also expressed the view that his inputs were not considered seriously by the employer. The employee explained:

RESEARCHER: How is the relationship with the employer? What about the hierarchy?

RESPONDENT: Employer usually never listens. They take ideas and use us for working like anything. They say that you are like a family member and we are working together, and they use us.

RESEARCHER: Do you mean they don't give credit?

RESPONDENT: Credit means, only when there is a product or application [that] comes into the market, patent or something comes, then credit. That is different. I am talking about things before that. They have to listen. I am not here without any knowledge.

Interaction with Academia

One of the important actors that is expected to aid in the innovation process is the academia. In order to understand the process through which such relationships are established and how they function in real time, the founders of the start-ups were asked to share their experience in case they had interacted with any academic institutes. Technically, since all the start-ups examined are located in a TBI, they are hosted by an academic institute and have a direct relationship in that sense. By virtue of their presence in the TBI, the start-ups get access to high-end machinery and laboratory space at the academic institutes at a subsidised price. However, in addition to that, there are other forms of relationships, such as technology licencing and sponsored projects. In the following discussion, it is examined how such arrangements are made between academic institutes and start-ups. Among the start-ups interviewed, except one, none of the firms had transferred any technology from an academic institute. Two firms had a joint project with academia. However, the start-up founders who interacted with academia expressed serious apprehensions and narrated negative experiences of their interaction. For instance, the founder of a start-up who had transferred technology from a CSIR institute named Institute for Chemical Technology (ICT) noted that through a common friend, he got to know about the availability of technology at ICT. He said that the technology that was licenced did not live up to what was promised by ICT. But the association with ICT has helped him secure BIG from BIRAC, an amount of Rs 50 lakh provided to early stage start-ups.

> So through a common friend of mine and ICT guys, I realised they have technologies relating to this. Spoke to them and they were very bullish, spoke big things like it's amazing and it would replace lot of established technologies and all that. But it was interesting and at that point of time, I just took a judgement call that we will go with this, it's a good idea. But the problem is, whatever they promised was not there. They vastly exaggerated. As [is] usually the case. But I was stuck. I already had paid them Rs 5 lakhs. The total deal was for Rs 10 lakhs. The area

was good and they let me work in their lab and stayed there for a year, worked with them and developed the project further. They had something which was only 5% ready to go to the market, but they said it's ready to go to the market. They say this all the time. When you go there, there is nothing much, very little. What helped me though was not their technology, ..., there was nothing. What helped me though was the name of the institute with which I went to BIG and said we have a partnership with ICT and it is a perfect example for Make in India, technology commercialisation from a national lab to a local entrepreneur and that's the way it clicked. It's a strategic play. I got something from them but it was definitely not technology. It was the name.

The terms and conditions of the agreement were such that the cost of the technology was Rs 10 lakh, with royalty sharing for three years at the rate of 3% on sales. But since the technology was not up to the desired levels for the founder of the firm and also since there were no sales immediately, the founder and the academic institution in question negotiated and arrived at a new contract. He said,

We had to pay royalties for three years. I paid them 50% including GST which went up to Rs 5.9 lakhs and when the time came for [the] next instalment I told them I am not going to pay you till I make sales. I didn't say that I will not pay anything. Still a positive relationship. I told them you have to support entrepreneurs, so wait for another one year may be till I start making sales. Then I will give you. The deal we had with them was 3% on sales as royalties for three years. They were helpful, but not in the way they should have been.

Explaining how the negotiation of agreements between academia and industry takes place, this founder who had a joint project with an academic institute stated the following.

We have to sit and see what is everybody's contribution. We calculate how much time we spent and how much time they spent. For example, you have a protein, first you identified it and you don't know how to take it and you don't know what to do to realise its potential. Then you come to me and I will use my technology to do it, since you identified and you are the inventor of that you will get [a] major share of the pie. The company involved in development activities will get lesser. But if the person has not identified and just has [a] theoretical idea and I do the whole work, then I will get the major part and he will get [the] small chunk.

However, almost all of the respondents felt that in India, academic institutes have less rigour and that the industry-academia linkage is very weak when compared with global institutions such as Stanford and the Massachusetts Institute of Technology (MIT).

> I think developing countries don't have the academic rigour. Well, this is completely off topic, but we don't have that professionalism. In India, the linkage between academia and industry is very weak. It should be strengthened and that too organically. Then it begins to make sense. Right now our standard is pretty low. So, you cannot expect to have good outcomes. See, look at Stanford and MIT, they both have added 2 trillion dollars to their economy each. Here our entire research ecosystem in terms of working on relevant problems which have application in health care, energy whatever is not worth it. So that element is not there in India. They don't understand the basics of the market, and they don't pick the right questions to answer.

Inter-firm Relationships

Most of the start-ups, especially in the biopharmaceutical sector, depend on other firms for a variety of services. These inter-firm relationships are established as a part of cost-cutting and also to focus only on the expertise that the start-up has. Some start-ups also provide CRO service in order to gain revenues, as well as to improve their own capabilities. A founder of a start-up explained the reasons for depending on other firms, saying that these relationships are important to bring the product to the market quickly rather than doing everything by themselves. He explained that this dependency on other firms would help them focus on their own strengths and the innovative aspect while allowing them to get the already established services at a cheaper price:

> See, what is important? Whether you want to have the molecule in the market quickly. Whether you want to exploit the market quickly, whether you want to explore more science quickly or whether you want to say I will do everything myself. What is it? Both are good. Both have their advantages and disadvantages. By outsourcing, we can do more science immediately. We can focus on our strengths. Or we will have to build all those strengths. We will have to get that expertise. You have to either train your own people or you have to get people who have that expertise. Now you can grow like that organically or you can instantly hand over, people will develop it and you can focus on your strengths again. Instead of trying to say that I will do everything. You can make them part of your team. Say for example you want to build a rocket. Say you have a breakthrough technology and breakthrough engine, you don't have to build the entire rocket yourself, right? You collaborate with people who can do it. You can look at it as a collaboration.

Some firms also perform CRO services for others, particularly to generate revenues, as well as to improve capabilities. A founder of a firm that performs CRO services explained that performing contract research for other organisations helped them in understanding the current industrial perspective and also helped them in earning some revenue:

> Actually it helps in knowing the current industrial perspective with regard to API[2] intermediates, how the industry thinks, and what is the commercial feasibility of a particular process. Even if it is a success in [the] R&D stage, it may not work that way when you scale up and when you go for further commercialisation. So there the thought process and economic perspective is [sic] very different. Even if a particular project is running almost in a slightly good manner, they may stop it. You get to know different thought processes and also earn some revenues.

Overall, it appears that inter-firm relationships play a crucial role in the functioning of MBT start-ups. According to the founders, these relationships are important for a variety of reasons. While in some cases they help in getting done the already established procedures at a cheaper price, some firms perform work for other firms so that they can earn some revenues and also get to understand the current trends in the industry.

Investment Practices and VC

The firms were also enquired about their source of investment and VC. The founders of 16 firms responded that their initial source of capital was either their own savings or they borrowed from their family or friends. Subsequently, 11 of them received a BIG grant from BIRAC as a source of seed capital and the rest of them are hoping to get it.

> [T]he thing with first-generation entrepreneurs is that we don't have much capital, all of us. We are not sitting with Rs 2–3 crores in the bank, mostly, most of the cases. If you have property, your dad is going to kill you if you sell that property. So that is not going to happen. So we have to start and play safe. Which is why most people should plan it properly. In my case, when I went to [the] Middle East to set up an incubator, with that I could make some bunch of money. Then I knew I could come out, plan something and start.

Except for three firms, none of the firms received VC, and no firm received VC at the seed-funding stage. The scenario reflects the general situation in the country where there is a lack of VC support for early stage MBT start-ups. The three firms that received VC funds did so only after they were able to establish the proof of concept (PoC). All three of the start-ups that received VC funding other than establishing a PoC also have their own IP assets. These IP assets provide investors real-time assurance to speculate and place safe bets on their investments. Looking at the social practices of valuation, Birch (2017) points out that the valuation of MBT firms is dependent on intangibles like patents, which act as income-deriving assets for these companies. It is based on this valuation that the investors invest in companies, which then the companies use and further raise the value of the companies, leading to their growth. The best-case scenario anticipated in such relationships is a successful exit strategy for the start-ups, which is either out-licencing their innovations or M&A by big pharmaceutical companies or IPOs.[3] The implications of the social practices of valuation are also witnessed from the narratives of those founders who received VC support. For instance, the firm which received VC funds, when asked about the process of pitching for investment, described the process as "very simple," saying that technology and their patent portfolios did everything.

> It was very simple; the technology and IP did everything. We gave a presentation and they liked it.

However, it also emerged from the interviews that there were instances where the founders of the firm declined an offer because it was felt that the investors were not contributing any value to the firm but were rather only interested in making returns on their investment.

> No. We are not doing that [pitching for VC]. We did one time, but it was a mistake. We have been shortlisted but we were not interested because they are not value-added investors.

Explaining what is meant by value-added investors, this founder said,

> Value-added investors mean[s] who can help your company to grow rather than take one part of the company and make ten times out of it? Not like that. He has to work with us. He should say, I will give Rs 1 crore, and I will be with you and I will see what can I bring to your company. So say that you need his contacts, he will introduce you [to] his contacts, this is kind of value-added investors.

In the case of firms that did not have a successful experience with VC funds, they responded that it wasn't difficult to pitch for investment given the virtue of their location in a TBI. However, what led to their failure was the stage of start-up, lack of IP assets, and tractions.

> Meeting an investor if you are in an incubator is not difficult. They will come with suits and all listen to all the guys. But in my case, they said that, you are too early and you do not have any tractions.[4]

DBT and BIRAC

The firms were also asked about their opinion on BIRAC and DBT. Almost all the firms expressed a positive opinion about BIRAC and identified it as an agency "that provides grant[s]." Except for one firm, none of the firms spoke about anything at great length except BIRAC's financial support. This is interesting given the fact that BIRAC provides various kinds of support, including investment, infrastructure, and institutional support. All of these start-ups have received/are receiving various kinds of support other than financial support from DBT. But both start-ups that received grants and start-ups that didn't receive them spoke very highly about BIRAC in terms of only financial support. However, there are also several firms which received funding but raised several issues with BIRAC. Interestingly, while some founders felt that the funding by BIRAC has to increase from the existing levels, others feel that BIRAC is too liberal in its funding.

> BIRAC is good by giving a little bit of money to establish. I appreciate them. But the thing is, a number of grants they are giving and the number of ideas India has, it's not enough. India has 1.3 billion people and they are spending Rs 300 million as grant[s]. You think, the proportion. That's the ecosystem. But since I got it, I should say it's good.

Several apprehensions also have been raised by the respondents about the selection procedure saying that the selection mechanism of BIRAC is dominated by academicians, and ideas that do not have commercial potential also get funded:

> Right now, actually, there are a lot of funding schemes available which are too liberal in giving funding. That's my opinion. All kind[s] of dumb ideas get funded in India. In fact, we should be a little bit more tight and rigorous. If you look at BIG and SPARSH and all these, the committee will be full of academics. What do academics know about markets commercially? They don't know anything. They like the idea, they like the science, they fund. Usually 99% of the BIG committee will be academics. Not industry people.

Exit Strategy and the Accumulation

Finally, the firms were asked about their exit strategy. All of the firms, specifically in the biopharmaceutical sector, responded mentioning out-licencing as their exit strategy, and a few (mostly medical device firms) of them wanted to scale up, manufacture, and market their products. The exit strategy of the firms particularly reflected a common practice across the globe, which is that of a small firm out-licencing to a big firm and earning licencing fee as well as a certain percentage of royalties based on sales. The exit strategy is also an example of the complex division of labour, where innovations brought out by the small start-ups are out-licenced to big firms as a part of the win-win strategy. But an important question that arises here is, what in case the innovation fails? It is now an established fact that 90% of start-ups fail (Patel, 2015). Given such a high rate of risk, this complex division of labour is a win-win for only a few start-ups. However, especially in the biopharmaceutical sector, this gives an opportunity for the big firms to cherry-pick the innovation without taking the same levels of risk and generate high revenues. The exit strategy of start-ups is also evidence of how double-layered accumulation takes place. All the biopharmaceutical firms interviewed for this study responded that their exit strategy is to out-licence their innovation to a bigger firm.

A member of a relatively successful biopharmaceutical firm explained their exit strategy as "so simple." The firm knows that it cannot manufacture biopharmaceuticals because it costs somewhere between Rs 100–200 crore. So the firm's exit strategy is to develop the technology and licence it to big firms.

> Exit strategy is so simple. Our exit strategy is to develop a technology and out-license. PoC was established even before we started the firm. We can't manufacture biosimilars because it is very expensive and require Rs.100–200 crores. We also thought that we can have a joint venture with other big companies.

Explaining why out-licencing is such a common exit strategy, the respondents mentioned that it is very difficult, for start-ups cannot afford to take the innovation to the market on their own.

> In life science, this is the only strategy because taking product into market takes a very long time. You take biopharma, diagnostics, and investments that are required for clinical trials or anything, you need huge investment. I don't think startups can really afford that. So they have to opt for out-licensing.

Based on these responses, the double-layered accumulation takes place in Indian MBT start-ups as follows. From the narrative of the founders of start-ups, it emerges that the most common source of initial seed capital is either BIRAC grants or individual savings and in some cases both. Following this in the growth stage, once the firms develop technologies to a desirable level, they approach for VCFs. With this investment (M_1), the start-ups come up with an innovation (C_1). Now the exit strategy of start-ups indicates that they want to out-licence their innovation to a big firm and then generate revenues (M'_1). This is the first layer of accumulation. This M'_1 is the capital investment by the big firm which licenced the innovation and by adding further value to the innovation markets the product or uses the innovation in their production process for cost-cutting and thereby extracts value (M_2). This is the second layer of accumulation. This double-layered accumulation is a specific phenomenon of knowledge economies where innovation and IPRs play a crucial role in economic activity. This is because here investment takes place for the same product by two different entities. While it may be argued that the complex division of labour by involving multiple business organisations takes place in a variety of economic activities—for example, in the case of IVCs, there are multiple organisations that are involved in a single production process—double-layered accumulation cannot take place there. In a typical economic activity involving multiple organisations, generally, different parts of the value chain are distributed among different organisations in the form of outsourcing. Here the economic logic at play is that these multiple organisations also make investments, but these investments are not to initiate an economic activity by themselves, but rather to perform outsourced work for multiple bigger firms and ensure returns on investment from all such work.

Further, there is a difference in market forms in which both of these economic activities take place. Both these economic activities involve two levels of market operations. One is for the small firm to involve itself with a bigger firm to ensure returns on investment, and the second is the bigger firm selling the final product in the market. The second level of market operation is largely similar for both these economic activities, while the difference lies in the first level of market operation. In the first level of market operation in which outsourced work takes place, for example, in the garment and textile sector, Kumar (2020) explains that, by virtue of the presence of multiple actors to perform the same outsourced work, there is an increase in the supply for a given demand which drives down the price of the work due to competition and thereby leading to what he calls *monopsony capitalism*. Due to this decreasing price of the outsourced work, the small business organisations may not necessarily entail a higher return on their investment from a single production process.

Now, if we take the case of out-licencing, here innovation is 'the single economic process' that determines the value, and the start-ups invest in this innovation that they themselves initiate—not outsourced to them by other firms—because of its market potential. Not to forget that this innovation is a monopoly of the start-ups because of the IPRs. Birch and Tyfield (2013) characterise this as "social expectations" of an asset-based market. It is with the help of IPRs that the first level of market operation takes place where start-ups out-licence their innovation. In this form of market activity, since the innovation is monopolised, supply is stagnant and demand drives the price of innovation—i.e. the higher the demand, the higher the price. However, the second level of market operation is to make this innovation reach the final consumer, which needs a further higher level of investment which the start-ups themselves do not possess and hence out-licence it to a bigger firm that can make such investments. The bigger firm also makes an investment that is based on the value of the innovation and its market potential, thereby leading to the double-layered accumulation. For the double-layered accumulation to take place, along with the complex division of labour, there is also a complex form of market activity, and hence it is a specific characteristic of knowledge-based economies.

In the following section, this process of double-layered accumulation is detailed more clearly through a case study of a relatively successful biopharmaceutical start-up named BW. In addition, the case of BW also helps to put in perspective how all the previously discussed elements discussed play a role in the accumulation process.

Start-Ups and Capital Accumulation in the MBT Sector— Case Study of BW

BW is a biopharmaceutical firm located at the TBI named Centre for Cellular and Molecular Platforms[5] (C-CAMP) in the Bangalore Life Science Cluster (BLiSc). BLiSc comprises C-CAMP; National Centre for Biological Sciences (NCBS), one of the most renowned life science research centres in India focusing on fundamental research; and the Institute for Stem Cell and Regenerative Medicine (InStem), a DBT autonomous research institute. The idea of this cluster is that all the elements of the cluster can work together in order to promote biotechnology innovation and entrepreneurship in India. C-CAMP was established in 2010, and BW was one of the first incubates here. BW is a spin-off of another firm named Cell-Works Research, headed by Dr. Anand Kumar, an NRI serial entrepreneur who returned from the US after working in the semiconductor industry (Kumar, 2017). Cell-Works is a subsidiary of Cell Works Inc. whose headquarters is based in San Francisco, US. It was started with an objective to use simulation processes implemented in semiconductors to understand biological mechanisms (Datta, n.d.). As one of the founding members recollects in an unpublished[6] essay (ibid.) penned down by himself, Cell Works had its initial collaboration with Astra Zeneca[7] to biologically validate their in-silico model of E.coli bacteria. The head of Astra Zeneca R&D then was Dr. Balasubramanian, and this project was headed by Dr. Shantanu Datta. It was this initial collaboration that later led to the formation of BW with Dr. Anand Kumar, Dr. Balasubramanian, and Dr. Shantanu Datta as its founding members. This initial estimate of the project was 50,000 USD for one year, according to details penned down by Datta (ibid.). Datta recounts that when this project was started, Dr. Anand Kumar had to deal with the "bureaucracy of a multinational corporate" for about six months. He explains that "most multinational pharma are weary of data leakage and hence have an army of expensive lawyers who try to ring fence everything related to intellectual property," and hence Kumar had to deal with the bureaucracy. Datta left Astra Zeneca after working there for 20 years and joined Cell Works to head the drug discovery arm. After

Datta moved to Cell Works, they started working on discovering an effective tuberculosis (TB) drug from a combination of previously used drugs.[8] For this project as well, Cell Works collaborated with Balasubramanian of Astra Zeneca. Balasubramanian, along with Cell Works, applied for a grant with the global philanthropic organisation Wellcome Trust and received a grant of one million USD. During this period, Cell Works got laboratory space from C-CAMP to run an experimental laboratory. One of the first employees recounted,

> When we started this company it was just this place (a single row of lab benches). I was embedded in Prof. Ramaswamy's lab and this was his lab and I was just part of this. That's how it started and then we evolved.
>
> (Source: Personal interview)

Prof. Ramaswamy was a professor at InStem and was also CEO of C-CAMP then. The collaboration for a TB drug brought out two combination treatments which were hitherto unknown and superior to the previous line of treatment according to Datta. Eventually, Balasubramanian also came out of Astra Zeneca in 2013 and joined Cell Works. After this in 2014, the Astra Zeneca research centre in Bengaluru got shut down, and at the same time, Cell Works also shifted its focus towards making oncology drugs, realising that the market potential in oncology drugs is much higher than that of drugs for infectious diseases. This led to the shutting down of the infectious diseases group at Cell Works.

Anand Kumar, along with Datta and Balasubramanian, started a new start-up named BW with a focus on infectious diseases at C-CAMP in 2014. The focus of BW is to develop drugs for superbugs. Superbugs are those infections which are antibiotic resistant and BW focuses on Gram $-$ve[9] infections. Most of the employees who work in BW have previously worked at Astra Zeneca and came to BW through persuasion by either Balasubramanian or Datta (Datta, n.d.). The CEO of the company is Anand Kumar. Among the founding members, it is only Anand Kumar who had previous experience working within a start-up ecosystem. This is largely due to his experience in the Bay Area of the US (Anand Kumar, 2017). Anand Kumar also specialises in cross-border investment, as well as the cross-border setting up of companies in India and the US (ibid.). He is also part of a team trying to create a Bangalore-Bay a Area corridor (ibid.) reminiscent of the Indo-US corridor created during the time of the software boom in India (Upadhyaya, 2004). Anand says the only thing that Bengaluru lacks is a VC ecosystem, and they are studying the Bay Area VC ecosystem in the US to replicate it in Bengaluru (ibid.). Anand Kumar is also a founding member of the Escape Velocity (EV) business accelerator, an accelerator focused on life science start-ups. EV has its business operations both in India and Singapore. Interestingly, three of the five founding members of EV own start-ups at TBIs sponsored by the government. In fact, the firms of two founding members of EV are still accessing subsided infrastructure at TBIs, while on the other hand, they have established their own private business accelerator. Anand Kumar is also an angel investor and invests in other business ventures (Anonymous, n.d.), while on the other hand, he seeks investment for his firm from other investors. The other two founding members, Datta and Balasubramanian, do not have a similar experience as Anand Kumar, other than spending a large part of their lives at a multinational pharmaceutical firm. This background also explains the division of labour among the founding members of the firm. While Anand Kumar is the CEO of the firm, involving himself mostly with the investments, Datta is the chief scientific officer and Balasubramanian is the chief operating officer and head of R&D of the firm. Currently, BW has nearly 20 employees. One of the founders explained that during the early days of the firm, all the employees settled for salaries below industrial norms; however, they were provided with employee stock options, taking inspiration from Infosys[10] (Datta, n.d.). The case of BW as a start-up also helps examine the aspect of hierarchy in start-ups. Balasubramanian explained the difference between working in a start-up and a multinational firm as follows:

> The big constraint [in MNC] was that it's highly process driven, highly bureaucratic. Decision making was a high-end constraint. Decision making was several layers removed from the action. So the big difference between a large company and startup, is the vibrancy in a startup, closeness to where the action is, everybody is also involved in the decision making. It is not several layers above. And so while some of the advantages of so-called "advantages of infinite resources" that we miss out of industry, I actually don't miss that. Because that is a mirage.... The startup environment for me is just a fantastic thing. Sometimes I ask myself, why didn't I do it much earlier in my life?
>
> (Balasubramanian, 2018)

However, he also admits that the industry background helps their firm phenomenally. His response to the question in an interview, "Does industry background help you?" was the following:

> [P]henomenally. I mean the industrial background is a massive, massive help. In fact, our success at Bugworks, yesterday Shantanu was saying that, "we acquired Astra Zeneca (AZ)". No, why he is saying that is because 50% of our staff is from AZ and all of the senior staff is from AZ. What we bring to the table is robustness, goal oriented, and in terms of the rigour that comes into the science. It is actually consistency and going towards the goal and phenomenal data rigour. That comes from the industry.
>
> (Ibid.)

Further, if we examine the organisation of the production process, it takes place through a network of organisations and outsourcing. Inside the BW office only strategy, risk-taking, decision-making and project management takes place, while execution and value addition takes place through outsourcing which includes hospitals, CROs. Etc. (Balasubramanian, 2019). This model of business according to its founder helps in keeping the capital costs low, human resource management minimal, and takes advantage of the expertise of the already established organisations (ibid.).

Another important component is the role of academia in this start-up. Technically, for being hosted at a TBI, BW gets access to the high-end infrastructure available at the academic institutions. While BW has academic collaboration with several institutions across the globe, it has very limited interaction with the academic institutions in the cluster (Bugworks, 2020). They had interaction with the professors from the academic institutes in the cluster initially and are planning to collaborate again by funding a project for a Cryogenic Electron Microscopic (Cryo-em) facility (source: personal interview). And recently, the BW website updated its academic collaborations page, saying that it is associated with Prof. S. Ramaswamy from InStem for a project on "Structural Biology of Targets Implied in Bugworks Drug Discovery" (ibid.). However, there was no technology transfer or presence of any faculty from the institutes in the Scientific Advisory Board (SAB) of BW. When the scientific head of BW was asked about the process through which this project would be funded, he said,

> You identify the experts in the field and talk to them. That's it. But C-CAMP also has mechanisms for this, but our collaboration is taking place at an individual level.
>
> (Source: Personal interview)

BW's success should also be largely attributed to the role of the state in setting up the biotech ecosystem in the country. Again in terms of investment and infrastructure, it received significant support from BIRAC and DBT. BW is housed at C-CAMP, which thereby gives them access to high-end equipment at NCBS and InSTEM, laboratory space at subsidised prices, and tax incentives for being a start-up. Explaining the role of DBT and BIRAC in BW, Anand Kumar, CEO of BW said,

> We are proud to partner with BIRAC. They have been supportive of early-stage, high-risk and high-innovation companies with unique methodologies. The government has been supporting very well, especially in the last 5 years. Without the DBT's support initially, Bugworks wouldn't exist today. The support was not just in terms of funding but also the much-needed infrastructure as well.
>
> (Gunashekar, 2016)

In terms of investment, BW received three grants from DBT after BW was officially incorporated. In 2014 itself, it received a BIG grant, as well as another grant under Biotechnology Industrial Partnership Programme (BIPP) from BIRAC. In 2016, again it was awarded a BIPP grant as a continuing grant. According to one of its founders, the firm received nearly Rs. 2.25 crores through grants from BIRAC. Explaining how this funding helped them, Balasubramanian said,

> DBT has been phenomenal for us. When we actually started Bugworks, we were a PowerPoint company basically. Right? We had a deck with very cute slides, we sold the fact that a bunch of us were coming from massive industry experience, we basically marketed that and it was on PowerPoint a promise and BIRAC funded us. We raised 2.25 crores and it was extremely healthy funding.
>
> (Balasubramanian, 2018)

Balasubramanian also explains the difference between grant funding from BIRAC and funding from investors such as VCs as follows:

> They [investors] take a company in proportion to whatever your valuation is to whatever the investment is irrespective of who the investor is [angel, VC, etc.]. Grant agency doesn't take any percentage ownership. Grant mechanism is non-equity based, non-diluted funding. The diluted funding irrespective of which basket it comes from, the principles remain the same. The percentage equity is commensurate to what we take is the value of the company to what amount of money is put in.
>
> (Ibid.)

BW had several types of investments. Along with grants from BIRAC, it had private investments in the form of angel investors and VCs. The company received two rounds of funding, pre-series-A and Series-A. In the pre-series-A round funding, the company raised almost 2.3 million USD in exchange of equity through the participation of several angel investors and VCs (Gunashekar, 2016). Kiran Mazumdar-Shaw, the CEO of Biocon, was also an angel investor of the firm. Other investors include Baxter Ventures and 3 one 4 Capital (BioSpectrum, 2017). Baxter Ventures is a corporate VC firm of Baxter International Inc, which is a Fortune 500 American healthcare firm (Fortune, 2019). Corporate VCs differ from institutional VCs in the sense that their investments go typically to the firms that work in an area similar to their interests. As one of the founders recalled, their first angel investment was serendipitous where a high-net-worth individual invested in them by taking a chance (source: personal interview). But, apparently, they made 200 presentations, almost all tailored differently to different investors, before they closed their pre-series-A (Balasubramanian, 2018). The company also had a Series-A round in 2018 where it raised nine million

USD, led by the University of Tokyo Edge Capital, Japan, Acquiphirma Holdings, 3 one 4 Capital, and other global and national angel investors (Economic Times, 2018). One angel investor who participated in this round is Shri Kumar Surya Narayan, who also heads another start-up at C-CAMP and is currently president of ABLE. From his experience, Balasubramanian shared the difference he observed between angel investors and VCs:

> We had more than 15 angels, but no one had gone out of the way and built a network for us including one of the later stage angels who was Kiran Mazumdar who invested in our company. Shri Kumar, he is a huge angel investor for us. In fact, he is the largest single angel investor for us. He has put so much of his personal money into the company. We get anecdotal connects here and there etc but not in an organised way. To be very honest, we do not have a very high expectation from that point of view because angels invariably are the people who we have just stumbled upon. It's not like we have actively sourced them. They come to know about us, they just get warmed by the cause and say, boom, I will put in money. VC, corporate investor, those are very different. Their clear objective is to lock in because it is not on a personal, you know, it basically is a business relationship and clear enough that they build their networks. Clear enough. It has also been a massive benefit for us in building networks.
>
> (Balasubramanian, 2018)

He went on to explain the constraints that come with VC investment:

> There [VC investment] it is all about extent of ownership, right? So when the investor's ownership when it exceeds a certain percentage of the company, they become part of the board. See, what runs a company finally is the board of the company, right? The investor whether it's a VC or an individual investor or a company investment when it starts exceeding a certain limit, typically when a particular investor starts creeping about 25% ownership of your company, they will be on your board. Then an equal voting right now. Is that a constraint? I don't know if it's a constraint but it's a structure. It can be a constraint because it depends on the individual who sits on the board. Now the individual because of the investor is more financially oriented as opposed to technology especially science based, then that mis-alignment can become very suffocating because a very financially oriented person always looks towards the bottom line which is, when is my return coming through, rather than actually pairing out the risk. So those are pluses and minuses.
>
> (Ibid.)

Another important aspect, the case of BW helps us understand is the critical role of IP in start-ups. BW holds IPR on four different patent families.[11] Explaining the importance of IP, Balasubramanian said,

We are an intellectual property based company and our *IP is our asset* [emphasis added]. We are looking at a hockey stick model, we either make it big or go six feet under and we are talking a year from now. If everything goes well, our asset is probably, you know, half a billion dollars' worth because it will be a first of its kind in about 50 years the [*sic*] mankind has seen. If it bombs, that's it.

(Balasubramanian, 2019)

In 2017, BW also received a grant worth 2.7 million USD from the global public-private accelerator CARB-X,[12] which funds projects on anti-microbial resistance drugs. Finally, BW has an exit strategy very similar to the established exit strategies of biopharmaceutical firms. The firm has already completed pre-clinical studies and animal trials and is planning to conduct Phase I trials sometime this year. After successful completion of Phase I, the firm plans to out-licence its molecules to a big pharma company and monetise them through royalties (ibid.). This exit strategy is common, especially in drug development start-ups because of the huge cost and infrastructural requirements to bring a successful drug to the market.

It is interesting how despite having such a rich background in terms of entrepreneurship and research, BW still chose this exit strategy. It is also an indication of the complex division of labour as a structural element in the biopharma sector. The case of BW is also clear evidence of how double-layered accumulation takes place. All the grants from BIRAC, CARB-X, and angel and VC investments (M_1) that BW secured are used to develop their innovation. The process of earning returns on this investment is through its exit strategy where BW is planning to out-licence its innovation (C_1) for a licencing fee and royalties (M'_1). The innovation (C_1) developed by BW also lets the company that licenced it generate returns on its investment (M_2) by adding further value and bringing the final product to market. This exit strategy exemplifies the double-layered accumulation, particularly in the case of successful biopharmaceutical firms—that is, very prominent globally right from the time of Genentech, the first successful biopharmaceutical start-up. This process ensures returns on investment for the VCs, the start-up founders, the employees who have stock options, and the bigger firm that licenced the innovation.

Notes

1 The GoI's JRF fellowship is a little bit higher than this.
2 Active pharmaceutical ingredients.
3 For a detailed discussion on VC operations, please see Zider, 1998; Hogarth, 2017.
4 Traction numbers indicate the existing customer base for the product.
5 C-CAMP is a TBI funded by the DBT.
6 The document was provided to the researcher by the author himself while conducting fieldwork.

7 The case of Astra Zeneca is discussed in detail in Chapter 3.
8 Four drugs—namely, Rifampicin, Ethambutol, Isoniazid, and Pyrazinamide—were being used to treat TB.
9 Bacteria are categorised into two types as Gram +ve and Gram –ve based on their structure.
10 Infosys is one of the first-generation IT firms in India that was successful.
11 All applications or filings of patents related to a single invention are considered a patent family.
12 CARB-X was launched in 2016 by government agencies in the US, the UK, and Germany in collaboration with private partners such as Wellcome Trust and the Bill and Melinda Gates Foundation (CARB-X, 2020).

Conclusion

The book is primarily concerned with understanding how the development of medical biotechnology (MBT) took place in India under a neoliberal political-economic system. The reason why this is an important concern to be addressed is because in the United States (US) where biotechnology first came into prominence, it took place through the coming together of several actors and institutions that were previously pursuing a conflicting set of agendas. Particularly, it was the state, academia, and finance capital that came together in the form of an ecosystem that in a way fuelled the biotech revolution in the US. The success of the biotech industry through this formation of an ecosystem in the US had two important implications for the rest of the world. One, the biotech innovation-business model in the US attained a kind of mythical status and was emulated by most countries. Second, under this innovation-business model, public institutions, particularly the state and academia, had to shed their social roles catering to the interests of a small section of the business class. The growth of this industry is the result of large-scale subsidies from the state that were implementing a neoliberal economic agenda at the same time as the implementation of austerity measures. State support for this industry in the US took place in various forms, such as direct monetary support, deregulation of financial markets, and enactment of favourable legislation, to list a major few. Of particular concern here is the legislation that transformed the nature of academic institutions from knowledge production as a common good to that actively encouraged towards knowledge commercialisation. The enactment of legislation such as the Bayh-Dole Act and the Stevenson Wylder Technology Transfer Act has set forward new goals for the academic institutions where commercialisation of knowledge became an important priority. The legislation allowed academic institutions to transfer research results that were federally funded to private industry. It was under such a climate that biotechnology as an economic opportunity started gripping the US. In fact, a substantial number of founders of biotech firms were professors from the academic institutions that made use of the public-funded research for private profit. The role of financial actors, particularly venture capitalists, is also significant in this process. After the deregulation of financial markets during the early 1980s and a reduction in capital gains tax, the volume of capital circulation in the form of venture capital (VC) substantially increased. One of the significant beneficiaries of this increased volume of capital is the biotech industry. While all of this discussion with respect to the US is critically looked at, what is missing from these debates is the Indian story which this book discussed. At the outset, it appears that the Indian biotech industry is on an upward trajectory with significantly increasing growth rates over the last three decades and aims to reach 100 USBD in revenue in the next few years. However, the story behind these increasing growth rates is the subject matter that this book has dealt with.

In India, the emergence of the biotechnology scenario began during the late 1980s at a time when the political-economic system of the country was transforming more towards a neoliberal way. As a result, the development of biotechnology in India right from its emergence was predicated on neoliberal principles. The Indian state realised the importance of biotechnology because of the prospects it had to offer for economic growth, and as a result, in the late 1980s, it devoted a generous set of resources for this purpose and ensured that necessary measures were taken for the growth of the MBT industry in India. It established a separate department for biotechnology (DBT), and India became the first country across the globe to have such a full-fledged DBT. Further, the early commercial endeavours of biotechnology in India also help us understand how the Indian state prioritised economic growth through private capital accumulation. In Chapter 1 of this book, this aspect has been discussed in detail by deploying the case studies of seven commercial endeavours in the MBT sector comprising public-sector units (PSUs), public-private partnerships (PPPs), and private-sector firms.

While the public-sector establishment in the name of BIBICOL was mandated to ensure self-sufficiency in vaccine production in India, it ended up as an agent to import vaccines manufactured by multinational companies (MNCs). This was the period during which PSUs were being discouraged and shut down as part of the neoliberal commitment of the Indian state. However, BIBICOL, despite its losses and inability to fulfil its initial mandate to produce vaccines indigenously, got to survive. This happened because BIBICOL was able to ensure profits to the MNCs for the sale of its vaccines at the behest of international organisations, such as the World Health Organization (WHO) and UNICEF. In the IVC of the vaccine market, the presence of BIBICOL helped MNCs to supply their vaccines in bulk to India, which BIBICOL then packaged and sold in the Indian markets. Similarly, the PPP initiatives in the early days were also only catering to the needs of the private industry. Two initiatives specifically discussed to demonstrate this are Genomed and TCGA. While Genomed is a case of a knowledge partnership that was based on the economic advantage the public-sector CSIR research institution could provide to the pharmaceutical firm NPIL, the case of TCGA was one where the private firm CMS exploited public resources for private profit.

In the case of private firms, the trajectory of four firms discussed in this study—namely, Biocon, ARCI, Shantha Biotechnics, and SLiSc—shows that these firms received significant support from the state for their success. The trajectory of Biocon is similar to the successful dedicated biotech firms in the US, which started with VC and private equity (PE) investments and then went public. While Biocon marked the birth of the first biotech billionaire in India, this growth largely took place through the 'managing of the state,' technology transfer from Cuban biotech firms, and serious disregard for organised local labour. The CEO of Biocon, along with several prominent industrialists, also established ABLE, a lobbyist organisation on behalf of the biotech industry with the state. In the case of ARCI, which is one of the very few research and development centres for multinational firms in India at that point in time, it was established because of the infectious disease market in India, as well as to take advantage of the low-cost human resources and infrastructure available in the country. This low-cost infrastructure and human resources were available to ARCI in the form of IISc, one of the most renowned public-funded scientific institutions in India. ARCI also led to the establishment of several biotech start-ups that provided it the prospects of acquiring them in order to expand its market. In the case of Shantha Biotechnics, it was established with underlying nationalistic rhetoric, with the help of the process patent regime, an angel investor from Oman, and with state support, developed a low-cost hepatitis B vaccine and made profits through a mass marketing strategy. Through this vaccine, Shantha Biotechnics challenged the monopoly of MNC firms in the Indian markets. However, in this battle for markets, ironically, despite Shantha Biotechnics' articulated concern for the nation that led to its establishment, it ended up being a subsidiary of an MNC through a process of mergers and acquisitions. Both ARCI and Shantha Biotechnics' initial association with a publicly funded academic institution met with dissent, indicating that such associations were unusual at that point in time. The case of SLiSc is the classic case of a scientific entrepreneur firm from IISc. The firm's trajectory provides evidence of the complex networks of production. SLiSc started as a platform firm, developing technologies that can be put to use by other firms. It also used to perform outsourced work for MNCs. In this process, SLiSc received significant VC and PE support, as well as several grants from the state. Through this capital, SLiSc later diversified its business in the US and India.

All the firms discussed here are successful first-generation MBT firms that were functioning without the presence of an organised ecosystem. Though the firms also received significant state support in India, an organised ecosystem, by bringing together all the necessary elements, took place only after 2007, when DBT started implementing its first national biotechnology strategy. With the implementation of this strategy, the MBT sector in India received huge support from the state in terms of increased budgets for DBT, infrastructure support, institution building, and capital support. Further, there was also an enactment of several favourable policies in related areas that are of direct interest to the MBT industry which was discussed in Chapter 2. With these initiatives, the biotech ecosystem in India came up in a big way, and currently, there are more than 2,600 biotech start-ups in the country, with two-thirds of them in the MBT sector, and this number is expected to go up to 10,000 by 2024 (BIRAC[a], 2019). The state support of the growth of the MBT industry is largely a part of its neoliberal commitment to provide supply-side incentives for private capital accumulation.

The book also examined the role of finance capital, particularly VC in Chapter 3. The theory of Biocapital that previously examined this question argued that there is no dominance of VC in India's MBT industry. However, available empirical evidence suggests that trend is changing over time with the deregulation of financial markets in India and also because of the exponential rise in the number of MBT start-ups in the country with the active role of the state. In fact, over the years, there is an overall increase in VC investments with higher growth rates. However, currently, the share of VC in MBT start-ups is low compared to that of other sectors. But there is no reason to believe that this situation is going to change. The overall growth of VC investments will also be reflected in the MBT sector because of the large-scale incentives provided by the state both to the investors and start-ups. While the provision of incentives helps in the reduction of risk for the investors, the exponential increase in the number of start-ups will have a direct impact on the number of firms entering the growth phase with reduced risk, which is a favourable environment for the investors. In this context, it is possible that the overall increasing investments in VC in the country will also spill over to the MBT sector.

Another important component of this ecosystem that is supposed to aid the growth of the MBT industry is academia. The literature that examined the question of the relationship between academia and industry in the US context tells us that it was with the advent of biotechnology that this relationship became prominent. However, in the Indian context—Chapter 4— the relationship between industry and academia existed right from the time of Independence. This is because publicly funded research organisations such as CSIR, as well as renowned public academic institutions such as IITs and IISc, engaged in industry-oriented research right from the beginning. Though there was no formal restriction on universities, universities largely stayed out of this kind of interaction. However, while the industry-academia relationship existed right from the beginning, the nature of this interaction changed over time. Between 1947 and 1991—i.e., from Independence to the economic reform period—the nature of the interaction between academia and industry was more of a demand-driven one. During this period, academia served the industry only on the basis of the existing demand. However, from 1991, with economic reforms taking place, the signing of the World Trade Organisation TRIPS Agreement, and the dominance of the knowledge economy and the primacy of patents, the nature of academia-industry interaction had started transforming. This was also the period during which biotechnology was rising to prominence in India. This transformation is reminiscent of the supply-side logic professed by the economic theories of neoliberalism. During this period, the state ensured that all necessary measures were put in place in the form of several policies in order to implement neoliberal reforms. In the neoliberal interaction, the interaction between academia and industry did not take place based on the current demand but rather on anticipating future demand. In this process, the academic institutes were encouraged to vigorously patent innovations, so much so that they became 'patent factories.'

However, this vigorous patenting in the anticipation of demand never really took fruition. This can be witnessed through the ratio of the number of patents licensed to the number of patents filed, which is abysmally low across all the institutions discussed in this study (CSIR, IISc, IITs, DBT autonomous institutes, and universities). This kind of vigorous patenting also led to a loss to the public exchequer. During this period, the state also focused on entrepreneurship, which is also one of the core tenets of the framework of neoliberalism. For this purpose, the publicly funded academic institutes were asked to encourage entrepreneurs through technology business incubators and scientific entrepreneurs by providing them with various kinds of subsidies. While during this period measures were taken to implement neoliberal reforms in the form of policymaking, there was largely no coercion on the institutions to implement the same. But since 2015, the state has started mandating scientists and publicly funded academic institutions to implement these neoliberal measures. The study notes that during this period, there was a complete transformation of the previously non-market-oriented academic value system into a corporate value system. Scientists are evaluated based on the number of patents and the amount of royalties they secure, the number of start-ups that they spin-off and mentor, etc., and universities are evaluated and granted autonomy based on their performance in successfully implementing these neoliberal measures. The justification provided by the state for the implementation of these coercive measures is that "COMMERCIAL success is the ONLY measure in long run" (emphasis original; MHRD, 2019, p. 21).

After examining the role of various actors and institutions in the growth of the MBT industry in India, the study attempted to understand how each of these actors and institutions played a role at the firm level through primary data collected from start-up founders and employees who worked in the start-ups (Chapter 5). In-depth interviews were conducted to understand the production process of the MBT start-ups in terms of the types of employment they provide, hierarchy and division of labour in the organisation, inter-firm relationships, investment practices, and exit strategies. From this exercise, it emerged that start-ups adopt a variety of employment practices, such as employing PhD students, providing employees with stock options, and, for a few of them, employees provided by public institutions such as

BCIL. The start-up founders projected these employment practices as more of a skill training for the employees which they argued would in turn help the individual research projects of the employers (for their PhDs or postdoctoral research) as well. However, it was found that such facilities and promises of training and self-development were effectively used to realise the goals of the firms. Most importantly, the restrictions they put on the employees in order to avail employment show that the avenues for personal growth for employees are limited in such firms. For example, in the case of a firm that employs students, while the founder says that these students will have an advantage in the labour market after their PhDs because of their industrial training, the students are not allowed to publish their research until they get a patent for the firm. These students are also not paid higher salaries but the same amount that the government of India pays a fellowship to the PhD students. Another founder generously mentions that he provides stock options to his employees, but the stock options are linked to commitment in terms of the number of years these employees work for the firm.

However, the work culture in start-ups is certainly less hierarchical and also there is no rigid division of labour, unlike in a corporate set-up. This opinion came out from both the employees and the employers. The start-ups also pointed to several inter-firm relationships in the form of outsourcing work to other firms or performing clinical research organisation (CRO) services for other firms. The start-ups engage with other firms for outsourcing in order to reduce the cost of production and also to only focus on the expertise. Through CRO services, the start-ups aim to earn revenues, as well as understand the current trends in the industry. When it comes to the question of investment, most of the founders started initially through their own savings or borrowings from friends and family. BIRAC also played a major role in providing investment to a large number of start-ups. However, it emerges from the discussion with the start-up founders that there is a dearth of VC investment as of now. Finally, the exit strategy of most of the biopharmaceutical start-ups is very similar and one that has been prominent for the last three decades, which is the out-licensing of innovation to another big firm. Through this exit strategy, it appears that start-ups are enabling what is called a *double-layered capital accumulation*, which is explained in Chapter 6.

Finally, the study concludes by noting that, while the advancements of science and technology (S&T) and innovation are critical aspects for social progress, these advancements are used merely for economic value extraction under the current (financial) capitalist system. It also appears that in instances when there is a conflict between the societal needs and economic value, in the current political economy set-up, the advancements of S&T will be put to use for the latter cause rather than the former. For example, during the recent COVID-19 crisis, several leaders of resource-poor nations raised serious apprehensions that patents on the potential COVID-19 vaccine would hamper the public health prospects of their nations. This is because governments such as that of the US have not yet fully committed to open science and innovation (*Nature*, 2020). During the recent World Health Assembly—the governing body of WHO—in 2020, when a resolution was proposed that any patents and information about the potential COVID-19 vaccines be pooled and shared with everybody in order to ensure equitable access to the vaccines, the US distanced itself from endorsing the proposal, saying that surrendering of intellectual property (IP) would stifle innovation. The CEO of Pfizer, one of the biggest pharmaceutical MNCs, called this proposal "nonsense" and "dangerous" (Newey, 2020). The CEO of another MNC Astra Zeneca stated, "I think IP is a fundamental part of our industry and if you don't protect IP, then essentially there is no incentive for anybody to innovate" (ibid.). Such apathy has been called out by *Nature*—one of the globally reputed science journals—in its editorial, saying that this situation is "unfortunate" (*Nature*, 2020). While this situation is definitely unfortunate, what led to this unfortunate situation is the crux of this study. And in order to avoid such unfortunate situations in the future, this study suggests that there needs to be a democratisation of science and its fruits put to use for the larger societal good in sharp contrast to the current monopolising tendencies.

References

AAAS. (2018). Research by Science and Engineering Discipline. https://www.aaas. org/programs/r-d-budget-and-policy/research-science-and-engineering-discipline. Retrieved February 15, 2019, from www.aaas.org.

AAAS. (n.d.). R&D at colleges and universities. https://www.aaas.org/programs/ r-d-budget-and-policy/rd-colleges-and-universities. Retrieved March 3, 2020, from www.aaas.org.

ABLE. (2020, March 29). Start-up corner. http://ableindia.in/startup/details/59. Retrieved March 29, 2020, from ableindia.in.

ABLE. (n.d.). *White paper on India's biotech startup ecosystem*. Bengaluru: Association of Biotechnology Led Enterprises.

Abrol, D. (2007). Publicly funded research and policy reforms in India: Lessons from the Council of Scientific and Industrial Research (CSIR). *Contemporary Perspectives*, *1*(2), 58–88.

Acharya, A. (2019, September). Direct-to-consumer genetic testing services gain a presence in India—Mapmygenome is bringing consumer genomics to a rapidly growing Indian population. (i. Inc, interviewer).

Acharya, R. (1995). *The impact of new technologies on economic growth and trade: A case study of biotechnology*. Netherlands: Maastricht University Press.

Aggarwal, A. (2001, June). Technology policies and technology capabilities in industry: A comparative analysis of India and Korea. *Working Paper – Indian Council for Research on International Economic Relations*, 1–48.

AIIMS. (2005). *Annual report*. New Delhi: All India Institute of Medical Sciences.

Ajay, D., & Sangamwar, A. (2014). Identifying the patent trend, licensing pattern and geographical landscape analysis of the Council for Scientific and Industrial Research (CSIR) of India between 2000 and 2011. *World Patent Information*, *30*(24), 1–8.

Alam, G., & Langrish, J. (1985). Government research and its utilization by industry: The case of industrial civil research in India. *Research Policy*, *13*, 55–61.

Anne, W. (2012). 23 and me blog. https://blog.23andme.com/news/announcements/announcing-23andmes-first-patent/. Retrieved March 23, 2020, from blog.23andme.com.

Anonymous. (n.d.). Our team. EVA. http://www.evaccel.com/our-team-founders. php. Retrieved June 12, 2020, from www.evaccel.com.

Anonymous. (1995a, July). Making research pay. *Economic and Political Weekly*, *30*(26), 1599.

Anonymous. (1995b, July 21). New rules push researchers close to biotech industry. *Science*, 269, 297–8.

Anonymous. (2001, November 10). Vision document on biotechnology. *Current Science*, 81(9), 1157.

Arora, A., & Bagde, S. (2007). The Indian Software Industry: The Human Capital Story https://papers.ssrn.com/sol3/papers.cfm?abstract_id=964465. Retrieved June 6, 2019, from papers.ssrn.com.

Arora, P. (2005). Healthcare biotech firms in India: Evolution, structure and growth. *Current Science*, 89(3), 458–63.

Arumugam, V., & Jain, K. (2012). Technology transfer from higher education institutions to industries in India—a case study of IIT Bombay. *Journal of Intellectual Property Rights*, 17(2), 141–51.

Athreye, S., & Chaturvedi, S. (2007). Industry associations and technology-based growth in India. *The European Journal of Development Research*, 19(1), 156–73.

Balasubramanian. (2018, May 5). Dr. Balasubramanian on Bugworks and biotech—Part 1. (CuriousCascade, interviewer). Available at https://www.youtube.com/watch?v=2q66Icf1I9s&t=460s

Balasubramanian. (2019, July 29). Startup journeys: Story of Bugworks Research India. *NMIMS Knowledge Series*. NMIMS Global Access-School for Continuing Education. Available at https://www.youtube.com/watch?v=mzZu2FJFIvk&t=1533s

Baru, R. (2003). Privatisation of health services—a South Asian perspective. *Economic and Political Weekly*, 38(42), 4433–7.

Basheer, S. (2016, May 17). An IP policy with no innovation. *The Hindu*.

Basheer, S., & Agarwal, P. (2017). India's new IP policy: A bare act? *The Indian Journal of Law and Technology*, 13, 1–26.

BCIL. (n.d.). Biotech industrial training programme. http://bcil.nic.in/bitp2019/index.asp. Biotechnology Consortium Industry Limited, Retrieved June 2, 2020, from bcil.nic.in.

Bernal, J. (1965). *Science in history—Volume 1*. Middlesex: Penguin Books Ltd.

Bharadwaj, A., & Glasner, P. (2009). *Local cells, global science: The rise of embryonic stem cell research in India*. London & New York: Routledge.

Bhardwaj, M., Naosekpam, A., & Tewari, R. (2017). Comparison of select Asian countries based on global S&T and education indicators. In R. Tiwari, *Industry-Academia R&D ecosystem in India: An evidence based study* (pp. 1–8). Chandigarh: Publication Bureau, Punjab University and Department of Science and Technology.

Bhargava, P.M. (1995, December 2). Biotechnology's decade of stagnation. *Economic and Political Weekly*, 30(48), 3049–50.

Bhargava, P. M. (2003, August 26). An extract from a textbook of history on planet Eurotopea in 2503. *The Hindu*.

Bhargava, P. M. (2009). Biotechnology in India: The beginnings. *Biotechnology Journal*, 4, 313–18.

Bhargava, P. M., & Chakrabarti, C. (1991, May). The role and present status of biotechnology in India. *Current Science*, 69(9&10), 513–17.

Bhattacharya, S. (2005). *Indian patenting activity in international and domestic patent system: Contemporary scenario*. New Delhi: Principal Scientific Advisor, Government of India.

Bhattacharya, S., & Arora, P. (2007). Industrial linkages in Indian universities: What they reveal and What they imply? *Scientometrics, 70*(2), 277–300.

BIBICOL. (n.d.). Milestones. http://bibcol.in/MILESTONES.html. Retrieved May 12, 2019, from bibicol.in. Bharat Immunological and Biological Corporation Limited.

Bielefeld, W., & Murdoch, J. (2004, June). The locations of nonprofit organizations and their for-profit counterparts: An exploratory analysis. *Nonprofit and Voluntary Sector Quarterly, 33*(2), 221–46.

BioSpectrum. (2003a, February 10). adVenture of Strand Genomics. *BioSpectrum.*

BioSpectrum. (2003b, March). Wanted a national biotechnology policy. *BioSpectrum,* pp. 1–5.

BioSpectrum. (2010, January 15). Why ain't biotech IPOs happening in India? *BioSpectrum.*

BioSpectrum. (2013, February 14). Strand receives investment from Burill & Company. *BioSpectrum.*

BioSpectrum. (2014, May 19). Is it curtains for Astra Zeneca R&D in Bangalore? *BioSpectrum.*

BioSpectrum. (2017, July 24). Bugworks Research & Pandorum Technologies grab top innovator award. *BioSpectrum.*

BioSpectrum (2019, June). BioSpectrum-top 20 biopharma companies. *BioSpectrum, 17*(6), 17–20.

BIRAC. (2015). *BIRAC 1st BIG report—2015.* New Delhi: Biotechnology Industry Research Assistance Council.

BIRAC. (2016). *Make in India for biotech: The way forward.* New Delhi: BIRAC.

BIRAC. (2020). Bioincubators nurturing entrepreneurship for scaling technologies. https://birac.nic.in/bionest.php. Retrieved April 2, 2020, from birac.nic.in.

BIRAC. (2020). Accelerating entrepreneurs (AcE) fund. https://birac.nic.in/aceFund.php. Retrieved April 2, 2020, from birac.nic.in.

BIRAC[a]. (2019). *India bioeconomy report—2019.* New Delhi: Biotechnology Industry Research Assistance Council.

BIRAC[b]. (2019). *India: The emerging hub for biologics and biosimilars.* New Delhi: Biotechnology Industry Research Assistance Council.

BIRAC[c]. (2019). *BIRAC innovation profiles—2018.* New Delhi: Biotechnology Industry Research Assistance Council.

Birch, K. (2006). The neoliberal underpinnings of the bioeconomy: The ideological discourses and practices of economic competitiveness. *Life Sciences, Society and Policy, 2*(3), 1–15. doi:10.1186/1746-5354-2-3-1.

Birch, K. (2017). Rethinking value in the bioeconomy: Finance, assetisation, and the management of value. *Science, Technology and Human Values, 42*(3), 460–90.

Birch, K. (2020). Technoscience rent: Toward a theory of rentiership for technoscientific capitalism. *Science, Technology and Human Values, 45*(1), 3–33.

Birch, K., Chiappetta, M., & Artyushina, A. (2020). The problem of innovation in techoscientific capitalism: Data rentiership and the policy of implications of turning personal digital data into a private asset. *Policy Studies,* 1–20. doi:10.1080/01442872.2020.1748264

Birch, K., & Tyfield, D. (2013, April). Theorising bioeconomy: Biovalue, biocapital, bioeconomics or what? *Science, Technology & Human Values, 38*(3), 299–327.

Blumenthal, D. (2003). Academic-industrial relationships in the life sciences. *The New England Journal of Medicine, 349*(25), 2452–9.

Blumenthal, D., Gluck, M., Louis, S. K., & Wise, D. (1986). Industrial support of university research in biotechnology. *Science*, 271(4735), 242–6.

Bowonder, B., & Mani, S. (2002). *Venture capital and innovation: The Indian experience*. Brussels: UNU/INTECH.

BugWorks. (2020, June 2). Academic Collaborators.https://bugworksresearch.com/partners/academic-collaborators/. Retrieved June 2, 2020, from bugworksresearch.com.

Business Line. (2000, November 9). Nicholas, CBT in pact for Genomed. *Business Line*.

Business Line. (2001, November 4). UTI Venture takes 17.5 pc stake in Strand. *Business Line*.

Business Line. (2004, September 7). Japanese co picks stake in Strand Genomics. *Business Line*.

Business Wire. (2010, October 1). Strand launches subsidiary Strand Scientific Intelligence, Inc. *Business Wire India*.

CAG. (2013). *Public private partnership for setting up the Centre for Genomic Application by Institute of Genomics and Integrative Biology. Comptroller and Auditor General of India*. New Delhi: CAG.

CARB-X. (2020, June 2). Funding Partners. https://carb-x.org/partners/funding-partners/. Retrieved June 2, 2020, from carb-x.org.

Chakma, J., Masum, H., Perampaladas, K., Heys, J., & Singer, P. A. (2011). Indian vaccine innovation: The case of Shantha Biotechnics. *Globalisation and Health*, 7(9), 1–10.

Chattopadhyay, D. (n.d.). IKP Knowledge Park. Presentation. Available at https://www.slideshare.net/amitkapoor/presentation-done-by-deepanwita-chattopadhyay

Chaturvedi, S. (2002). Status and development of biotechnology in India: An analytical overview. RIS discussion paper (28).

Chaturvedi, S. (2007, September). Indian innovation system and emergence of biopharmaceutical sector: Issues and prospects. RIS discussion paper (124).

Chaudhari, S. (2018, September). Impact of product patents on pharmaceutical market structure and prices in India. *Indian Institute of Management Calcutta-Working Paper Series* (813), 1–50.

Chial, H. (2008). DNA sequencing technologies key to the Human Genome Project. *DNA Sequencing Technologies Key to the Human Genome Project*, 1(1), 219.

Chibber, V. (2003). *Locked in place: State-building and late industrialization in India*. Princeton and Oxford: Princeton University Press.

CII, & Sathguru Management Consultants. (2017). *Biotech startups in India: At the cusp of global impact*. New Delhi: Confederation of Indian Industries and Sathguru Management Consultants.

Clarke, A. E., Shim, J., Shostak, S., & Nelson, A. (2009). Biomedicalising genetic health, diseases and identities. In P. Atkinson, P. Glasner, & M. Lock, *The handbook of genetics & society: Mapping the new genomic era* (pp. 21–40). London: Routledge.

Cooper, M. (2008). *Life as surplus: Biotechnology and capitalism in the neoliberal era*. Seattle: University of Washington Press.

Cromwell Schmisseur LLC. (2013). *Information and observations on state venture capital programs*. Washington: Department of the Treasury. Available at https://www.treasury.gov/resource-center/sb-programs/Documents/VC%20Report.pdf

CSIR. (1996). *Vision document—2001*. New Delhi: Council for Scientific and Industrial Research.

CSIR. (2009, November). *Encouraging development and commercialisation of inventions and innovations: A new impetus. Office memorandum.* New Delhi: Council for Scientific and Industrial Research.

CSIR. (2011). *CSIR @ 80: Vision & Strategy 2022.* New Delhi: Council for Scientific and Industrial Research.

CSIR. (2016). *Creation of CSIR innovation fund: Office memorandum.* New Delhi: Council for Scientific and Industrial Research.

CSIR. (n.d.). CSIR Milestones. https://www.csir.res.in/achievement/csir-milestones. Retrieved May 3, 2019, from www.csir.res.in.

Das, D. R., Kumar, M. S., & Mishra, A. Industry-academia interaction: Bridging the gap for the benefit of Society. In R. Tewari, *Industry-Academia R&D Ecosystem in India: An Evidence Based Study* (pp 260–9). Chandigarh: Publication Bureau, Punjab University and Department of Science and Technology.

Das, R. J. (2015). Critical observations on neoliberalism and India's new economic policy. *Journal of Contemporary Asia, 45*(4), 715–26.

Datta, S. (n.d.). *The Journey of Bugworks in the Quest for New Antibiotics.* Unpublished.

DBT. (2005). *National biotechnology Development strategy-I.* New Delhi: Department of Biotechnology.

DBT. (2012). *Indian biotechnology: The Roadmap to Next Decade and Beyond.* New Delhi: Department of Biotechnology.

DBT. (2015). *National biotechnology development strategy 2015–20.* New Delhi: Department of Biotechnology.

DBT. (2016). *Annual report 2015–16.* New Delhi: Department of Biotechnology.

DBT. (2018). *Expression of Interest (EOI) for Academic Institutions/Universities/ Research Institutions/Scientific Organizations/Section 8 Companies to Set Up New/to Upgrade the Existing Technology Transfer Offices.* New Delhi: Department of Biotechnology. Retrieved December 12, 2019 from http://dbtindia.gov.in/sites/default/files/EoI_TTO_Dec_2018.pdf

DBT. (2019a). About us. https://www.globalbioindia.com/aboutus.php. Retrieved December 12, 2019, from www.globalbioindia.com.

DBT. (2019b). *National biotechnology parks scheme.* New Delhi: Department of Biotechnology.

DBT. (2020, March 31). Biotech Science Clusters.http://dbtindia.gov.in/schemes-programmes/research-facilities-resources-technology-platforms/biotech-science-clusters. Retrieved March 31, 2020, from dbtindia.gov.in.

DBT. (n.d.-a). Department of Biotechnology-Key Statistics. http://dashboard.dbtindia.gov.in/. Retrieved February 12, 2020, from dbtindia.gov.in.

DBT. (n.d.-b). Introduction. http://dbtindia.gov.in/about-us/introduction. Retrieved May 13, 2019, from dbtindia.gov.in.

DBT. (n.d.-c). Patent Facilitation. http://dbtindia.gov.in/schemes-programmes/trans-lational-industrial-development-programmes/patent-facilitation. Retrieved April 5, 2020, from dbtindia.gov.in.

DBT. (n.d.-d). *Instructions for technology transfer and intellectual property rights. Annexure-V.* New Delhi: Department of Biotechnology.

Demain, A. L. (2010). History of industrial biotechnology. In W. S. Vandamme, *Industrial biotechnology. Sustainable growth and economic success.* Weinheim: WILEY-VCH Verlag GmbH & Co. KGaA.

Desai, A. V. (1980). The origin and direction of industrial R&D in India. *Research Policy, 9,* 74–96.

Deshpande, N., & Nagendra, A. (2017, July). Patents as collateral for securitization. *Nature Biotechnology, 35*(6), 514–16.

Dhanjal, S. S., & Sarkar, P. (2016, February 18). PE/VC fund managers cheer move to allow pension funds to invest in AIFs. *Live Mint.*

Differding, E. (2017). The drug discovery and development industry in India—two decades of proprietary small-molecule R&D. *ChemMedChem Reviews, 12,* 786–818.

DIPP & DBT. (2017). *Biotechnology sector: Achievements report. Make in India.* Department of Industrial Policy Promotion and Department of Biotechnology, Government of India.

Dorbian, I. (2018, October 9). PE backed Strand Life Sciences to buy Quest Diagnostics India medical diagnostics business. https://www.pehub.com/2018/10/pe-backed-strand-life-sciences-to-buy-quest-diagnostics-india-medical-diagnostics-business/#. Retrieved May 12, 2018, from www.pehub.com.

Dossani, R. (1999, October). Venture Capital and Innovation: The Indian Experience. Report of a Conference. Asia Pacific Research Center & Stanford University.

DST. (1974). *Research and development statistics 1973–74.* New Delhi: Department of Science and Technology.

DST. (2018). *National expenditure on research and development by sector.* New Delhi: Department of Science and Technology.

DST. (n.d.). Venture Capital Funds. http://tdb.gov.in/venture-capital-funds/. Retrieved December 20, 2019, from tdb.gov.in. Department of Science and Technology.

Economic Times. (2016, March 9). Government announces labour law exemptions for startups up to three years. *Economic Times.*

Economic Times. (2018, August 13). Bugworks Research bags Rs 62 crore in Series A. *Economic Times.*

Editorial. (1999, December). Conflict of interest. *Current Science, 77*(11), 1381.

Emmett, A. (2000, July 23). The human genome. *The Scientist.*

Englander, E. J. (1991). The political economy of biotechnology: Innovation and politics in an emerging industry. *Business and Economic History, 20,* 136–41.

Etzkowitz, H. (2003). *MIT and the rise of entrepreneurial science.* London and New York: Routledge.

Etzkowitz, H. (2013). Anatomy of the entrepreneurial university. *Social Science Information, 52*(3), 486–581.

Fan, P., & Watanabe, K. N. (2008). The rise of the Indian biotech industry and innovative domestic companies. *International Journal Technology and Gloabilisation, 4*(2), 148–69.

Feisee, L. (2002). Biotech in northeast Ohio conference—the role of the private sector in biotechnology: Research and development. *Health Matrix: The Journal of Law—Medicine, 12*(2), 357–65.

FICCI, Federation of Indian Chamber of Commerce. (2015). *Biotechnology landscape in India.* Federation of Indian Chamber of Commerce.

Financial Express. (2013, September). APIDC-VCL arm to invest Rs 8 cr in 3 biotech startups. *Financial Express.*

Fochler, M. (2016). Beyond and between academia and business: How Austrian biotechnology researchers describe high-tech startup companies as spaces of knowledge production. *Social Studies of Science, 46*(2), 259–81

Fortune. (2019). Baxter International. https://fortune.com/fortune500/2019/baxter-international/. Retrieved April 12, 2020, from www.fortune.com.

Foucault, M. (2003). *The birth of clinic*. London: Routledge.

Frankel, F. (2005). *India's political economy 1947–2004* (2nd ed.). New Delhi: Oxford University Press.

Frost & Sullivan. (2016). *2025 roadmap for India Biotech Industry*. New Delhi: Confederation of Indian Industries (CII).

Galambos, L., & Sturchio, J. L. (1996). The pharmaceutical industry in the twentieth century: A reappraisal of the sources of innovation. *History and Technology*, *13*(2), 83–100.

genomeWeb. (2005, September 1). Strand Genomics changes name to Strand Life Sciences. *genomeWeb*. Retrieved April 2018 from https://www.genomeweb.com/archive/strand-genomics-changes-name-strand-life-sciences.

George, S., Chandran, A. B., Nadh, P., & Apurva, K. (2017). Is drug development in India responsive to the disease burden? A public health appraisal. *Economic and Political Weekly*, *53*(30), 50–7.

Ghose, T., & Bisaria, V. (2000). Development of biotechnology in India. *Advances in Biochemical Engineering/Biotechnology*, *69*, 88–124.

Ghosh, D. (2014, July 21). Strand life sciences: Bringing genetic tests to the average customer. *Forbes India*.

Ghosh, P. (1996, November). Indian experience in commercialising institutionally developed biotechnologies. *Journal of Scientific and Industrial Research*, *55*, 860–72.

GoI. (2016a). *Startup India action plan*. New Delhi: Government of India.

GoI. (n.d.-a). Biotechnology. http://www.makeinindia.com/sector/biotechnology. Retrieved March 24, 2017, from www.makeinindia.com: http://www.makeinindia.com/sector/ biotechnology. Government of India

GoI. (n.d.-b). Venture funding support. https://www.startupindia.gov.in/content/sih/en/compendium_of_good_practices/angel_and_venture_funding.html. Retrieved April 2, 2020, from www.startupindia.gov.in. Government of India.

GoI. (2006). *Technology innovation and venture capital*. New Delhi: Planning Commission, Government of India.

GoI. (2009). *National knowledge commission—Report to the nation 2006–2009*. New Delhi: Government of India.

GoI. (2016b). *National intellectual property rights policy: Creative india; innovative India*. Department of Industrial Policy and Promotion. New Delhi: Government of India.

Gonzalo, M., & Kantis, H. (2017). Venture capital in India: A critical view from an evolutionary and systemic perspective. *15th International Globelics Conference*. Athens.

Gulifeiya, A., & Aljunid, S. M. (2012). Development of health biotechnology in developing countries: Can private-sector players be the prime movers? *Biotechnology Advances*, *30*(6), 1589–1601.

Gunashekar, R. (2016, January 29). Hottest startup: Soldiers against drug resistance terror. *BioSpectrum*.

Gupta, A., Bhojwani, H., & Koshal, R. (2000). Managing the process of market orientation by publicly funded laboratories: The case of CSIR, India. *R&D Management*, *30*(4), 289–96.

Gupta, S. (2015). Patenting activity in India in the post-WTO Era: With special reference to major scientific agencies in India. *PhD thesis*. Retrieved April 2020 from http://hdl.handle.net/10603/38909. Shodhganga.

Hackett, J. E. (2014). Academic capitalism. *Science, Technology and Human Values*, *39*(5), 635–8.

Harvey, D. (2005). *A brief history of neo-liberalism*. New York: Oxford University Press.

Hood, L., & Rowen, L. (2013). The Human Genome Project: Big science transforms biology and medicine. *Genome Medicine*, *5*(9), 1–8.

Indian Patent Office (n.d.). Patent Search Result. https://ipindiaservices.gov.in/PublicSearch/PublicationSearch/PatentSearchResult. Retrieved November 10, 2019, from ipindiaservices.gov.in.

Hogarth, S. (2017). Valley of the unicorns: Consumer genomics, venture capital and digital disruption. *New Genetics and Society*, *36*(3), 260–72.

Huggett, B. (2014). Reinventing tech transfer: US university technology transfer offices are adopting new models in search of increased return on research investment. *Nature Biotechnology*, *32*(12).

Huggett, B. (2017, March). Top US universities, institutes for life sciences in 2015. *Nature Biotechnology*, *35*(3), 203.

Huggett, B. (2018). Bringing up baby. *Nature Biotechnology*, *36*(5), 393–401.

Hughes, S. S. (2001). Making dollars out of DNA: The first major patent in biotechnology and the commercialization of molecular biology, 1974–1980. *Isis*, *92*(3), 541–75.

Hughes, S. S. (2011). *Genentech: The beginnings of biotech*. London: University of Chicago Press.

IBEF. (2017, May). Biotechnology. https://www.ibef.org/download/Biotechnology-May-2017.pdf. Retrieved May 1, 2018, from www.ibef.org: https://www.ibef.org/download/Biotechnology. India Brand Equity Foundation, Department of Commerce, Government of India.

IBEF. (n.d.). Pharmaceuticals. https://www.ibef.org/pages/17158. Retrieved July 2, 2018, from www.ibef.org. India Brand Equity Foundation, Department of Commerce, Government of India.

IGIB. (n.d.-a). About. http://admin.igib.res.in/aboutigib.html. Retrieved May 4, 2019, from igib.res.in.

IGIB. (n.d.-b). Home. https://www.igib.res.in/. Retrieved May 13, 2019, from www.igib.res.in.

IISc. (2017). Entrepreneurship. https://www.iisc.ac.in/entrepreneurship/. Retrieved on May 12, 2019 from iisc.ac.in.

IISc. (2019). Home. http://csic.iisc.ac.in/. Retrieved November 1, 2019, from iisc.ac.in.

IISc. (2018). Patenting at IISc. *Report*.

IIT Delhi. (2019, December 26). News. http://www.iitd.ac.in/content/iit-delhi-files-150-ips-2019-highest-ever-year. Retrieved February 12, 2020, from iitd.ac.in.

Jayaraman, K. (2001, April). India's biotech budget hiked. *Nature Biotechnology*, *19*, 299.

Jayaraman, K. (2005, April 7). India's strategy to bridge the public-private divide. *Bioentrepreneur, Nature*.

Joseph, R. K. (2015). *Pharmaceutical industry and public policy in post-reform India*. New Delhi: Routledge.

Joshi, A. (2017). Provocation, precedence and innovation: How Shantha Biotechnics shaped India's biotech future. In *Indian science transforming India – Impact of science in independent India: An anthology* (pp. 118–40). New Delhi: Indian National Science Academy.

Kalra, A. (2019, November). https://www.startupindia.gov.in/content/sih/en/reources/startup_india_notes/regulations_and_policies/corporate_social_responsibility_funding_incubators.html. Retrieved on April 12, 2020, from startupindia.gov.in.

Kharbanda, V. (2004). Changing structure of scientific communities in the 1990's. In V. Kharbanda, *Formation Growth and Changing Structure of Scientific Communities in India and China*. PhD thesis available at http://shodhganga.inflibnet.ac.in/jspui/handle/10603/16764.

Khokhar, M., & Tewari, R. (2017). Industry-academia R&D regimes in IITs. In R. Tewari, *Industry-Academia R&D Ecosystem in India: An Evidence Based Study* (pp. 82–137). Chandigarh: Publication Bureau, Punjab University and Department of Science and Technology.

Kleinman, D. L., & Vallas, S. P. (2001). Science, capitalism, and the rise of the "knowledge worker": The changing structure of knowledge production in the United States. *Theory and Society*, 30(4), 451–92.

Kohli, A. (2006). Politics of economic growth in India: 1980–2005—Part I. *Economic and Political Weekly*, 41(13), 1251–9.

Konde, V. (2009). Biotechnology business models: An Indian perspective. *Journal of Commercial Biotechnology*, 15(3), 215–26.

Krimsky, S. (2003). *Science in the private interest: Has the lure of profits corrupted biomedical research?* Maryland: Rowman & Littlefield Publishers.

Krishna, V. (2001). *Reflections on the changing status of academic science in India.* 231–46. Blackwell Publishers and UNESCO.

Krishna, V. (2007). Large public research systems: India's CSIR, the CNRS in France and the CSIRO. *Innovation: Management, Policy and Practice*, 9(2), 192–202.

Krishna, V., Patra, S. K., & Bhattacharya, S. (2012). Internalisation of R&D and globalisation of innovation: Emerging trends in India. *Science, Technology and Society*, 17(2), 165–99.

Kumar, A. (2017, November 17). Anand Anandkumar—entrepreneur speaker series at UC Berkeley. *Entrepreneur Speaker Series*. Available at https://www.youtube.com/watch?v=DiYunnN6Jhw

Kumar, A. (2020). *Monopsony capitalism: Power and production in the twilight of the sweatshop age.* New Delhi: Cambridge University Press.

Kumar, N. (1987). Biotechnology in India. *Development: Seeds of Change* (special issue on biotechnology), 4, 51–6.

Lee, D. P., & Dibner, M. D. (2005, July). The rise of venture capital and biotechnology in the US and Europe. *Nature Biotechnology*, 23(6), 672–6.

Lehman, V. (2010). Doing good by doing well? The political economy of the medical biotechnology in the United States. PhD thesis. UMI Dissertation Publishing.

Loeppky, R. (2005). History, technology, and the capitalist state: The comparative political economy of biotechnology and genomics. *Review of International Political Economy*, 12(2), 264–86.

Madhavi, Y. (2005). Vaccine policy in India. *PLoS Medicine*, 2(5), 387–91.

Madhavi, Y. (2007). Transnational factors and national linkages: Indian experience in human vaccines. *Asian Biotechnology and Development Review*, 9(2), 1–43.

Madhavi, Y. (2013). Vaccines and vaccine policy for universal health care. *Social Change*, 43(2), 263–91.

Madhavi, Y. (2014, June 14). Manufacture of consent? Hepatitis B vaccination. *Economic and Political Weekly*, 38(24), 2417–24.

Maiti, S. (2013). Council of Scientific and Industrial Research, and national planning, 1947–1958. *Proceedings of the Indian History Congress*, 74, 1019–24. Indian History Congress.

Marx, K. (1887). *Capital: A critique of political economy* (Vol. 1). Moscow: Progress Publishers.

Mashelkar, R. (2004). Restructuring of public R&D institutions: New challenges and opportunities. *Presentation*. Retrieved October 15, 2019 from http://web. worldbank.org/archive/website01503/WEB/IMAGES/MASHELKA.PDF

Medical Laboratory Observer. (2014, March 28). Strand Genomics and BioHealth Innovation partner to expand Strand Centers for Genomics and Personalized Medicine. *Medical Laboratory Observer*. Available at https://www.mlo-online. com/home/article/13006270/strand-genomics-and-biohealth-innovation-partner-to-expand-strand-centers-for-genomics-and-personalized-medicine

Merton, R. K. (1973). The normative structure of science. In N. W. Storer, *The sociology of science: Thereotical and empirical investigations*. Chicago: Chicago University Press.

MHRD. (2019a). *Atal ranking of institutions on innovation achievements*. New Delhi.

MHRD. (2019b). *Institution's innovation council*. New Delhi

MHRD. (2019c). *National innovation and startup policy 2019 for students and faculty*. New Delhi.

Ministry of Commerce. (2019). List of operational SEZ of India as on 31.03.2018. https:// commerce.gov.in/writereaddata/UploadedFile/MOC_636983712222577837_ LS-10-07-2019.pdf. Retrieved April 5, 2020, from commerce.gov.in.

Mirowski, P. (2012). The modern commercialization of science is a passel of Ponzi schemes. *Social Epistemology*, 26(3–4), 285–310.

Mishra, R. (2001, February 22). Draft plan to revive Bharat Immunologicals. *Business Line*.

Morini, C., & Fumagalli, A. (2010). Life put to work: towards a life theory of value. *Ephemera* (3/4), 234–52.

Morrison, C., & Lähteenmäki, R. (2017, July). Public biotech in 2016—the numbers. *Nature Biotechnology*, 35(7), 623–9.

Muzaka, V. (2018). *Food, health and the knowledge economy: The state and intellectual property in India and Brazil*. London: Palgrave Macmillan.

Mytelka, L. K. (1999). *Competition, innovation and competitiveness in developing countries*. Development Centre. Organisation for Economic Cooperation and Development.

Naidu, N. Chandrababu. (2000). *Plain speaking*. With Sevanti Ninan. New Delhi: Viking.

National Human Genome Research Institute. (n.d.). What is the human genome project? https://www.genome.gov/human-genome-project/What. Retrieved May 12, 2019, from https://www.genome.gov/: https://www.genome.gov/human-genome-project/ What

National Science Foundation. (1982). *University-industry research relationships: Myths, realities and potentials*. Washington, DC: National Science Foundation.

Nature. (2006, July 13). Is India's 'patent factory' squandering funds? *Nature News, 442*.

Nature. (2018, October 25). New head of Indian research giant to tackle funding issues and red tape. *Nature*.

Nature. (2020, May 21). Everyone wins when patents are pooled. *Nature, 581*(7808), 240.

Navarro, V. (2007). Neoliberalism as a class ideology; or the poltical causes of growth of inequalities. *International Journal of Health Services, 37*(1), 47–62.

NCL. (2019). Milestones. http://www.ncl-india.org/files/AboutNCL/History Milestones/1990_1999.aspx. Retrieved November 10, 2019, from ncl-india.org. Pune: National Chemical Laboratory.

NDTV. (2017). Clinical trials in India: Saving or risking lives? *We the People*. NDTV.

Newell, P. (2007). Biotech firms, biotech politics: Negotiating GMOs in India. *The Journal of Environment & Development, 16*(2), 183–206.

Newey, S. (2020, May 29). WHO patent pool for potential Covid-19 products is 'nonsense', pharma leaders claim. *The Telegraph*.

Nightingale, P., & Martin, P. (2004). The myth of biotech revolution. *Trends in Biotechnology, 22*(11), 564–9.

NIRF. (2016). University. https://www.nirfindia.org/univ. Retrieved March 2, 2019, from www.nirfindia.org. National Institute Ranking Framework.

NITI Aayog. (2015). *Report of the expert committee on innovation and entrepreneurship*. New Delhi: NITI Aayog.

OECD. (2009). *The bioeconomy to 2030: Designing a policy agenda*. Paris: OECD Publishing. https://doi.org/10.1787/9789264056886-en.

Office of Adviser to the Prime Minister—Public Information Infrastructure & Innovations. (2011). *University innovation clusters*. New Delhi: Draft Concept Paper.

Owen, R., North, D., & Bhaird, C. M. (2019). The role of government venture capital funds: Recent lessons from the U.K. experience. *Journal of Strategic Change, 28* (1), 69–82.

Padmanabhan, G. (2003, September). Growth of biotechnology in India. *Current Science, 85*(6), 712–19.

Patel, N. (2015, January 15). 90% of startups fail: Here's what you need to know about the 10%. *Forbes*.

Patnaik, P. (2016, July). Economic liberalisation and the working poor. *Economic and Political Weekly, 51*(29), 47–51.

Pisano, G. (2006). Can science be a business? Lessons from biotech. *Harvard Business Review, 84*(10), 114–24.

Planning Commission. (1951). Scientific and industrial research. In P. Commission, *1st plan document*. New Delhi.

Planning Commission. (1956). Scientific and technological research. In P. Commission, *2nd five year plan*. New Delhi.

Planning Commission. (1992). 8th five year plan (Vol-2). *Plan Document*.

Planning Commission. (2006). *Working group report on strengthening academia industry interface (including public private partnership)*. New Delhi: Planning Commission of India.

Prasad, V. (2019, April 19). Reason behind Shantha Biotechnics start? Hybiz TV. Available at https://www.youtube.com/watch?v=AWGsuKJ8kXA

Principal Scientific Advisor. (2019). *R&D expenditure ecosystem: Current status and way forward*. New Delhi: Office of Principal Scientific Advisor, Government of India.

Principal Scientific Advisor. (n.d.). *Strategic options for commercialisation of patents in India*. New Delhi: Office of the Principal Scientific Advisor.

Pulakkat, H. (2015, November 27). How allowing professors to start companies triggered red-hot startup labs. *Economic Times*.

Puliyel, J., & Madhavi, Y. (2008). Vaccines: Policy for public good or private profit? *Indian Journal for Medical Research*, 127(1), 1–3.

Quadria Capital. (2018, February). Quadria Capital invests in India's leading specialized diagnostics firm Strand Lifesciences. https://www.quadriacapital.com/quadria-capital-invests-in-indias-leading-specialized-diagnostics-firm-strand-lifesciences2/#:~:text=Singapore%20%2F%20New%20Delhi%2C%20%5B8th,integrated%20and%20specialized%20diagnostic%20company. Retrieved September 2018 from quadriacapital.com

Radder, H. (2010). The commodification of academic research. In H. Radder, *The commodification of academic research: Science and the modern university* (pp. 1–23). Pittsburgh: University of Pittsburgh Press.

Rai, J. (2016, January 29). Strand Life Sciences to list on NASDAQ via Reverse Merger. *VC Circle*. Available at https://www.vccircle.com/strand-life-sciences-get-listed-nasdaq-through-reverse-merger/. Retrieved September 2018 from vccircle.com

Rai, J. (2018a, January 4). HCG combines clinical lab services unit with Strand Life Sciences. *VC Circle*. Available at https://www.vccircle.com/hcg-combines-clinical-lab-services-unit-with-strand-life-sciences/. Retrieved September 2018 from vccircle.com.

Rai, J. (2018b, February 8). Quadria Capital backs Strand Life Sciences. *VC Circle*. Available at https://www.vccircle.com/quadria-capital-backs-strand-life-sciences/. Retrieved September 2018 from vccircle.com

Raina, D. (2006). Science since independence. *India International Centre Quarterly*, 33(3/4), 182–95.

Ramachandran, J. (1991a, May 25). Strongly goal oriented biomedical research - Astra Research Centre India. *Current Science*, 60(9&10), 533–6.

Ramachandran, R. (2000, September 2). A comprehensive programme. *Frontline*, 17(18).

Ramachandran, R. (2008, March 29). Ailing policy. *Frontline*, 25(7).

Ramachandran, S. (1991b). Government funding and support—the department of biotechnology. *Current Science*, 60(9&10), 518–23.

Ramakrishnan, N. (2016, April 4). The science of tapping talent. *Business Line*.

Ramani, S. V. (2002). Who is interested in biotech? R&D strategies, knowledge base and market sales of Indian biopharmaceutical firms. *Research Policy*, 31(3), 381–98.

Ramani, S. V., & Maria, A. (2005). TRIPS: Its possible impact on biotech segment of the Indian pharmaceutical industry. *Economic and Political Weekly*, 40(7), 675–83.

RBI. (2016, October 20). Investment by a foreign venture capital investor (FVCI) registered under SEBI (FVCI) regulations, 2000. *RBI Circular*. India: Reserve Bank of India. Available at https://www.rbi.org.in/scripts/NotificationUser.aspx?Id=10649&Mode=0

Reddy, P. (2012, March 28). CSIR spends a whopping Rs. 74.24 crores on securing patents in India & abroad; refuses to disclose revenues from patent licensing. https://spicyip.com/2012/03/csir-spends-whopping-rs-7424-crores-on.html. Retrieved November 10, 2019, from spicyip.com.

Reddy, P., & Sigurdson, J. (1997). Strategic location of R&D and emerging patterns of globalisation. *International Journal of Technology Management*, 14(2–4), 344–61.

Reddy, Y. (1998, August). Speeches and Interviews. https://www.rbi.org.in/scripts/BS_SpeechesView.aspx?Id=265. Retrieved April 7, 2020, from www.rbi.org.in.

Rediff. (2000, November 8). NPIL, CBT tie up for GenoMed. *Rediff Business News*. Available at https://www.rediff.com/money/2000/nov/08genome.htm. Retrieved August 2018 from rediff.com.

Reid, S. E., & Ramani, S. V. (2012). The harnessing of biotechnology in India: Which roads to travel? *Technological Forecasting and Social Change*, 79(4), 648–64.

Report of the third reviewing committee of scientific and industrial research. (1965). *Minerva*, 3(3), 356–84.

Rose, N. (2001). The politics of life itself. *Theory Culture and Society*, 18(6), 1–30.

Rose, N. (2007). *The politics of life itself*. Princeton: Princeton University Press.

Roth, C. R. (2000). *From Alchemy to IPO: The business of biotechnology*. Cambridge: Perseus Publishing.

Roy, V. (2017). *The Financialization of a Cure: A Political Economy of Biomedical Innovation, Pricing and Public Health*. University of Cambridge. PhD thesis.

Sabarinathan, G. (2017). *Venture capital and private equity investing in India—an exploratory study*. Indian Institute of Management (IIM) Bengaluru, working paper (542).

Sabberwal, G. (2006, May). New pharma-biotech company formation in India. *Nature Biotechnology*, 24(5), 499–501.

Saberwal, G. (2013). Giving voice to India's entrepreneurs. *Nature Biotechnology*, 31(2), 104–8.

Saberwal, G. (2016). India's intellectual property-based biomedical startups. *Current Science*, 110(2), 167–71.

Sandhya, G., Jain, A., & Mathur, P. (1990, December 22). S and T planning, policy directions and CSIR. *Economic and Political Weekly*, 25(51), 2800–5.

Scoones, I. (2003). Making policy in the "new economy": The case of biotechnology in Karnataka, India. IDS Working Paper (196).

SEBI. (1999). *Report of KB Chandrasekhar Committee on Venture Capital*. Mumbai: Securities and Exchange Board of India.

SEBI. (2003). *Advisory Committee on Venture Capital under Dr. Ashok Lahiri*. Mumbai: Securities and Exchange Board of India.

SEBI. (n.d.-a). Registered Venture capital Funds. https://www.sebi.gov.in/sebiweb/other/OtherAction.do?doRecognisedFpi=yes&intmId=21. (S. a. India, Producer) Retrieved June 2020 from www.sebi.gov.in.

SEBI. (n.d.-b). Registered Foreign Venture Capital Investors. https://www.sebi.gov.in/sebiweb/other/OtherAction.do?doRecognisedFpi=yes&intmId=25. (S. a. India, Producer) Retrieved June 2020 from www.sebi.gov.in.

SEBI. (n.d.-c). Investment details of VCF/FVCI https://www.sebi.gov.in/statistics/investment-details-VCF-FVCI.html. Retrieved March 29, 2020, from www.sebi.gov.in.

Sen, S., & Smith, H. L. (2008). Science, institutions and markets: Developments in the Indian biotechnology sector. *Regional Studies*, 42(7), 961–75.

Shantha Biotechnics. (n.d.). http://shanthabiotech.com/about-us/history-milestones/. Retrieved May 4, 2019, from shanthabiotech.com.

Shapin, S. (2008). *The scientific life: A moral history of late modern vocation*. Chicago and London: University of Chicago Press.

Sharma, D. C. (2015). *The outsourcer: The story of India's IT revolution*. Cambridge, Massachusetts: The MIT Press.

Sheth, A., Krishnan, S., & Samyuktha, T. (2020). *Indian venture capital report 2020: Perspectives on the funding and startup ecosystem*. Bain and Company, Indian Venture Capital Association.

SID. Society for Innovation and Development, IISc (n.d.). About. https://sid.iisc.ac.in/about/. Retrieved May 2, 2019, from sid.iisc.ac.in.

SIDBI. (2019). *Private investing in India—Venture capital focus: State of sector report*. New Delhi: Small Industrial Development Bank of India.

Singh, B. (1986, August 23). Reviewing the CSIR. *Economic and Political Weekly*, *21*(34), 1511–18.

Singh, B. (1987, April). Perspective before CSIR. *Economic and Political Weekly*, *22*(17), 752–6.

Singh, S. (2016). *Myth Breaker: Kiran Mazumdar-Shaw and the Story of Indian Biotech*. Noida: Harper Collins.

Slaughter, S., & Leslie, L. L. (2001). Expanding and elaborating the concept of academic capitalism. *Organisation Overview*, *8*(1), 154–61.

Slaughter, S., & Rhoades, G. (2004). *Academic capitalism and new economy: Markets, state and higher education*. Baltimore: John Hopkins University Press.

SLiSc. (2013, December 5). Strand Center for Genomics and Personalized Medicine.

SLiSc. (n.d.-a). Bioinformatics. https://strandls.com/bioinformatics/. Retrieved May 4, 2019, from strandls.com.

SLiSc. (n.d.-b).Strand Laboratory Locations. https://strandls.com/strand-laboratory-locations/. Retrieved May 8, 2019

SLiSc. (n.d.-c). https://strandls.com/strand-life-sciences-us/. Retrieved May 2, 2019, from www.strandls.com.

SLiSc. (n.d.-d). The Avadis platform. https://www.strand-ngs.com/avadis-platform. Retrieved May 1, 2019, from www.strand-ngs.com.

Smith, L. C. (2014, May–June). Patenting genes: What does Association for Molecular Pathology V. Myriad Genetics mean for genetic testing and research. *Public Health Reports*, *129*, 289–92.

Smith, S. B.-S. (2008). Science, Institutions, and markets: Developments in the Indian biotechnology sector. *Regional Studies*, *42*(7), 961–75.

Somasekhar (2000, September 27). Indo-Russian vaccine project: Focusing on new formulae. *Business Line*.

Srivastava, P., & Chandra, S. (2012). Technology commercialization: Indian university perspective. *Journal of Technology Management and Innovation*, *7*(4), 121–31.

Stern, S. (1995). Incentives and focus in university and industrial research: The case of Synthetic Insulin. In N. Rosenberg, A. C. Gelijns, & H. Dawkins, *Sources of medical technology: universities and industry-medical innovation at the crossroads* (Vol. V, pp. 157–87). Washington, DC: National Academy Press.

Sunder Rajan, K. (2005). Subjects of speculation: Emergent life sciences and market logics in the US and India. *American Anthropologist*, *107*(1), 19–30.

Sunder Rajan, K. (2002). Biocapital: The constitution of post genomic life. PhD thesis. Massachusetts: MIT Press.

Sunder Rajan, K. (2003). Genomic capital: Public cultures and market logics of corporate biotechnology. *Science as Culture*, *12*(1), 87–121.

Sunder Rajan, K. (2006). *Bio Capital: The constitution of post genomic life*. Durham: Duke University Press.

Sunder Rajan, K. (2007, May–June). Experimental values: Indian clinical trials and surplus health. *New Left Review*, *45*, 67–88.

Sunder Rajan, K. (2012). The capitalization of life and the liveliness of capital. In K. S. Rajan, *Lively capital: Biotechnology, ethics and governance in global markets* (pp. 1–44). Durham and London: Duke University Press.

Sunder Rajan, K. (2017). *Pharmocracy: value, politics and knowledge in global biomedicine*. Hyderabad, Telangana, India: Orient Black Swan.

Sunder Rajan, K., & Leonelli, S. (2013). Introduction: Biomedical transactions, postgenomics, and knowledge/value. *Public Culture*, *25*(3), 463–75.

Surana, K., Singh, A., & Sagar, A. (2018). *Enhancing S&T based entrepreneurship: The role of incubators and public policy*. New Delhi: Department of Science and Technology.

TCG Life Sciences Limited. (2007, September 28). *Draft red herring prospectus*. India: TCG Life Sciences Limited.

The Hindu. (2019, September). Now, India Inc can deploy CSR funds on research. *The Hindu*.

Tilak, J. B. (2014). Private higher education in India. *Economic and Political Weekly*, *49*(40), 32–8.

Times of India. (2016, October 19). CSIR wants labs to stop random filing of patents. *Times of India*.

Tiwari, R. (2017). Industry-academia programmes/schemes of public and private sectors. In R. Tiwari, *Industry-academia R&D ecosystem in India* (pp. 12–81). Chandigarh: Publication Bureau, Punjab University and Department of Science and Technology.

UGC. (2015). *UGC guidelines for establishing university-industry inter-linkage centres in universities*. New Delhi: University Grants Commission.

UGC. (2018, February 12). Categorisation of Universities (Only). New Delhi.

UGC. (2019, July). List of all universities. https://www.ugc.ac.in/oldpdf/consolidated%20list%20of%20All%20universities.pdf. Retrieved November 10, 2019, from ugc.ac.in.

Upadhyaya, C. (2004). A new transnational capitalist class? Capital flows, business networks and entrepreneurs in the Indian software industry. *Economic and Political Weekly*, *39*(48), 5141–51.

Vallas, S. P., & Kleinman, D. L. (2008). Contradiction in convergence: Universities and industry in the biotechnology field. *Socio Economic Review*, *6*(2), 283–331

Valluri, S. (1993). CSIR and technological self-reliance. *Economic and Political Weekly*, *28*(14), 565–8.

Venture Center. (n.d.). http://venturecenter.co.in/vips.php. Retrieved June 1, 2020, from venturecenter.co.in.

Viale, R., & Etzkowitz, H. (2010). *The capitalization of knowledge: A triple helix of university-industry-government*. Cheltenham and Northampton: Edward Elgar.

Vijay Raghavan, K. (2016). As India's economy grows, we will have more support for science. *Biotechnology: An Agent for Sustainable Socio-Economic Transformation*. (A. Bhatta, Interviewer) Nature Publishing Group.

Visvanathan, S. (1998). A celebration of difference: Science and democracy in India. *Science*, *280*(5360), 42–3.

Viswajanani, S. (2019, July 9). CSIR initiatives—technology development and licensing, and the evolving paradigm. *Presentation*. Downloaded from http://apctt.org/sites/default/files/VJS_HRDC_Technology_Commercializatiion.pdf

Zider, B. (1998, November–December). How venture capital works. *Harvard Business Review*.

Ziman, J. (1996, August 29). Is science losing its objectivity? *Nature, 382,* 751–4.

Index

Pages in *italics* refer figures; **bold** refer tables and pages followed by n refer notes.

ecosystem 115; finance capital role 56; funds, *see* VC funds; Indian state and 63–4; industry 12, 61, 63; investment 119–20; investor 57; and MBT in India, *see* VC and MBT in India; number and value of deals, 2008 and 2018 62, 62; State Small Business Credit Initiative 64n3; theory of Biocapital 57–8, 64
venture capitalism 57

Well Spring Hospital 28–9, 42n2
World Bank (WB) 61
World Health Assembly 128
World Health Organization (WHO) 25–7, 37, 39, 123, 125
World Trade Organisation (WTO) 54
World War I 5
World War II 5, 66

Yusuf Bin Alwai Abdullah, H. E. 38

For Product Safety Concerns and Information please contact our EU
representative GPSR@taylorandfrancis.com
Taylor & Francis Verlag GmbH, Kaufingerstraße 24, 80331 München, Germany